MENTAL HEALTH SERVICES

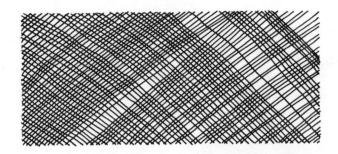

—Edited by—
Paul B. Pedersen
Norman Sartorius
Anthony J. Marsella

MENTAL
HEALTH
SERVICES

The Cross-Cultural Context

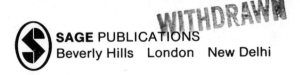
SAGE PUBLICATIONS
Beverly Hills   London   New Delhi

For information address:

SAGE Publications, Inc.
275 South Beverly Drive
Beverly Hills, California 90212

SAGE Publications India Pvt. Ltd.
C-236 Defence Colony
New Delhi 110 024, India

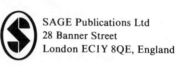

SAGE Publications Ltd
28 Banner Street
London EC1Y 8QE, England

Printed in the United States of America

Library of Congress Cataloging in Publication Data

Main entry under title:

Mental health services.

   (Sage series on cross-cultural research and methodology; v. 7)
   Includes bibliographies.
     I. Psychiatry, Transcultural. 2. Mental Healing.
I. Pedersen, Paul, 1936-   .   II. Sartorius, N.
III. Marsella, Anthony, J.   IV. Series: Cross-Cultural
research and methodology series ; 7.
RC454.4.M46 1984   362.2   83-26945
ISBN 0-8039-2259-0

FIRST PRINTING

Contents

To Anne Pedersen, Vera Sartorius, and Joy Marsella,
for all their help and support.

About the Series

The Sage Series on Cross-Cultural Research and Methodology was created to present comparative studies on cross-cultural topics and interdisciplinary research. Inaugurated in 1975, the series is designed to satisfy a growing need to integrate research method and theory and to dissect issues in comparative analyses across cultures. The recent ascent of the cross-cultural method in social and behavioral science has largely been due to a recognition of methodological power inherent in the comparative perspective; a truly international approach to the study of behavioral, social, and cultural variables can be done only within such a methodological framework.

Each volume in the series presents substantive cross-cultural studies and considerations of the strengths, interrelationships, and weaknesses of its various methodologies, drawing upon work done in anthropology, political science, psychology, and sociology. Both individual researchers knowledgeable in more than one discipline and teams of specialists with differing disciplinary backgrounds have contributed to the series. While each individual volume may represent the intergration of only a few disciplines, *the cumulative totality of the series reflects an effort to bridge gaps of methodology and conceptualization across the various disciplines and many cultures*.

We take pleasure in adding *Mental Health Services: The Cross-Cultural Context* to the series. The coeditors of this volume, Paul Pedersen, Norman Sartorius, and Anthony Marsella, are key scholars in the cross-cultural understanding of psychopathology, counseling and psychotherapy, and the delivery of mental health services. Pedersen and his coeditors have enlisted the aid of thirteen other experts to prepare chapters. Some chapters concern substantive areas that are critical in conceptualizing and implementing various aspects of mental health services in culture-specific regions or cultures, while other chapters deal with the need to understand the nature of certain conditions (e.g., schizophrenia) or certain processes (e.g., interviewing and assessment) that may be viewed as culture general. This book is a valuable addition to the growing literature on counseling and therapy from an international perspective. By adding it to the series we believe that a genuine and important contribution to this aspect of cross-cultural research and methodology has been made, much to the benefit of the growing international community of mental health workers and professionals.

—Walter J. Lonner
Western Washington University
—John W. Berry
Queen's University

Preface

Traditional systems of mental health services have a cultural bias favoring dominant social classes that can be counterproductive to an equitable distribution of services. This book is intended to increase the visibility of indigenous mental health traditions, to challenge the potential ethnocentrism in their unwarranted use by providers. The constructs of "healthy" and "normal" that guide the delivery of mental health services are not the same for all cultures and might betray the culturally encapsulated counselor.

This book is organized according to the emic (culture-specific) and etic (culture-general) approaches to mental health services. The most basic question a mental health service provider must ask in a culturally different setting is "When do you adapt the assessment, diagnosis, and therapy methods of a dominant culture and when do you substitute the unique approach of an indigenous culture? This book is directed toward answering that question. The combined chapters will provide a useful and valuable framework for matching a mental health service delivery plan with culturally different clients.

In the last decade, mental health professionals have been urging more attention to cultural issues. In more recent times, accreditation of programs in psychiatry, psychology, social work, and other professions has begun to require and enforce specific curricula in cross-cultural issues. In addition to formal classroom instruction, there are increased opportunities for cross-cultural study through in-service programs. This book is an attempt to help meet the growing demand for a cross-cultural approach. We hope that these chapters communicate the enthusiasm and commitment we feel toward this book.

We would like to acknowledge the contributions of persons who have assisted us in preparing this book. Thanks go to Rebecca Cole-Turner and Karen Slick for helping to proofread the manuscript, to Bonnie Ozaki for assembling the index, to Pat Moran for facilitating communications among the editors through innumerable letters and photocopies, and to our friends at Sage who have supported our idea for this book since its inception. As Series Editors, Walt Lonner and John Berry provided valuable guidance in the refinement of our book. The variety of other support staff who assisted the editors and authors of this book are also gratefully acknowledged.

—Paul B. Pedersen
Norman Sartorius
Anthony J. Marsella

1

INTRODUCTION
The Cultural Complexity
of Mental Health

PAUL B. PEDERSEN

The basic problem facing mental health diagnosis and service providers is how to describe behavior in terms that are true to a particular culture while at the same time comparing those behaviors with a similar pattern in one or more other cultures. When the perspective of one culture, such as the Euro-American Western tradition, is *imposed* on another culture the result is a "pseudoetic" (Triandis, 1977) or an "imposed etic" (Berry, 1975). However, without a framework for comparison there can be no communication. Even Pike (1966), in his original conceptualization of this dichotomy, suggested that the two elements not be treated as a rigid dichotomy, but as a way of presenting the same data from two viewpoints. Since that time others have assumed that we need emic items to measure etic constructs (Triandis, 1977) and approaches that combine the emic and etic approaches are widely used in the social sciences (Trimble, Lonner, & Boucher, 1983). Berry (1975) suggests that we enter a culture with and through an *imposed etic* and then gradually modify our outside perspective toward a *true emic* perspective. Those etic elements not eliminated by emic considerations form a *derived etic,* based on empirical data from the specific culture as well as general patterns.

There is increased pressure for the providers of mental health services to acknowledge the importance of their consumers' cultural environment. Not only are mental health service providers ethically committed to be interculturally skilled, but their responsibility for accuracy and effectiveness also demands that they account for cultural complexity in mental health services (Atkinson, Morton, & Sue, 1979; Favazza & Oman, 1977; Marsella & Pedersen, 1981;

Marsella & White, 1982; Pedersen, Draguns, Lonner, & Trimble, 1981). Increased interest in cultural alternatives for mental health services have resulted from changes in the political, social, and economic power balance of the world community, a need for more cost-effective alternatives than one-to-one therapy, increased inter-action between Western and non-Western cultures, and a more comprehensive understanding of how mental health is affected by environmental networks.

THE IMPORTANCE OF COMPLEXITY

The effective therapist will generate several alternative interpreta-tions and understandings of an event to reflect the complexity of environmental factors influencing the event. There is a tradition that favors complicated explorations, including the principle of comple-mentarity (Bohr, 1950), theories of cognitive complexity (Harvey, Hunt, & Schroder, 1961; Schroder, Driver, & Streufert, 1967), and theories of adult development (Fowler, 1981; Gilligan, 1982; Kegan, 1982; Kohlberg, 1969; Lovinger, 1976; Perry, 1970). This literature assumes that persons who are more cognitively complex are more capable, that cognitive complexity is related to an advanced level of development, and that many phenomena can best be understood if several different "complementary" perspectives are applied to them. This principle has been applied to a number of different disciplines, including economics, political science, gastroenterology, eclesiology, literary criticism, the philosophy of science, and organizational behavior (Bartunek, Gordon, & Weathersby, 1983).

Complexity involves two processes that are "complementary" to one another. Differentiation is the ability to perceive several dimen-sions in a stimulus array. Integration is the development of complex connections among differentiated characteristics. The cognitively complex person can perceive multiple dimensions of an event while simultaneously applying one or more classification systems to describe the phenomena. Persons with higher levels of cognitive complexity can take another person's perspective (Triandis, 1977), demonstrate less prejudice (Gardner, 1972), make moral judgments on the basis of principle through reciprocal role taking (Kohlberg, 1969), and are better able to resolve conflicts cooperatively (Eise-man, 1978). Persons at earlier stages of personality development tend to be concrete, sterotypic, and dogmatic, while more advanced stages involve complex, abstract, and more precise and specified thinking styles.

Just as differentiation and integration are complementary processes, so are the emic (culture-specific) and etic (culture-general) perspectives necessarily interrelated. The terms "emic" and "etic," borrowed from phonemic and phonetic analysis in linguistics describing the rules of language, imply a separation of general and specific cultural aspects. Although research on the usefulness of emic and etic categories has been extensive (Lonner, 1980; Berry, 1980; Brislin, 1983), the notion of a "culture-free" (universal) etic has been just as elusive as the notion of a "culture-pure" (totally isolated) emic in the complexity of cross-cultural relationships. Increased attention to special interest psychologies related to age, lifestyle, socioeconomic statis, gender, and an assortment of formal, nonformal, or informal affiliations have complicated cultural identity and have introduced a multicultural definition described by Andre (1981) as "multicultural research methodology."

This chapter is written from the perspective of the "outside expert" having to enter a strange and unfamiliar culture to provide an appropriate mental health service and an accurate diagnosis. What would that outside expert need to know? How could the expert escape from imposing an outside (etic) perspective? One of the first questions a service provider confronts in an unfamiliar culture is whether to work from a more familiar "foreign" perspective brought in from the outside or learn a new or less familiar "local" perspective on mental health and illness. The culture-general (etic) and more familiar perspective may provide a useful entry point into the culture providing that the outsider is willing to modify generalizations to fit the reality of the culture-specific (emic) situation. The outsider becomes a mediator by looking at culture-general and culture-specific examples of mental health services. This book will attempt to balance the importance of each for the *mediation* of a mental health service.

Each of the chapters in this book emphasizes either a culture-general or a culture-specific perspective. The "general" chapters focus primarily on a technique, method, or treatment going across cultures. The "specific" chapters focus primarily on specific populations describing the cultural context of mental health services. A concluding chapter synthesizes guidelines and observations that integrate both specific and general perspectives. While there are many techniques, methods, or treatments not included in this book, just as there are many additional populations not mentioned, the chapters will build on these selected examples to demonstrate our point. Both the general and specific perspectives are important.

CULTURE-GENERAL APPLICATIONS

The first section of this book examines five examples of culture-general applications for mental health. In Chapter 2, Juris Draguns points out ways that a visitor's observations are complicated by variations in the cultural perspectives of both the host and the visitor. How is behavior that is disturbed and pathological differentiated from behavior that is culturally characteristic? The very criteria of an outside assessment bring implicit cultural assumptions to the new and unfamiliar setting. How is psychopathology differentiated from deviance when pathology is only a small portion of deviance? Patterns of deviation in each culture are extremely complicated, especially when viewed from the perspective of an outsider. How does one avoid confounding the effects of the observer, the setting, and the community with those of the culture and/or the disorder? The problems of accurate assessment in an unfamiliar culture arise from the need to interpret the same event from the cultural perspectives of both the host and the observer. Draguns proceeds to answer these questions in the light of new methodologies and scientific instrumentation, to identify those tasks that have been left unfinished and those problems that need to be solved in the future.

Scientific advances in processing data on symptom-based measures have increased the reliability of diagnosis. The objectification and standardization of symptom checklists, interview schedules, and systematic measures of negative affect have helped to clarify patterns of similarity through a more precise methodology. There has also been a corresponding increase in the sophistication of technology for translating verbal messages through the use of special English and a more accurate translation of terms describing subjective emotional states. The translation process includes attention to the form as well as the content of the message being translated, where the observer him- or herself becomes the instrument of assessment.

Draguns explains both the emic and the etic strategies for assessment. According to the etic strategy for cross-cultural differences, the emphasis is more on the quantitative than the qualitative, where pan-cultural similarities overshadow differences. According to the emic strategy, the emphasis has been largely on descriptions of exotic symptoms in particular cultures. Draguns discusses a strategy proposed by Marsella (1980) to proceed from an emic identification, quantity the data, and draw etic conclusions through comparison. This intergration of emic and etic perspectives provides a possible avenue for making emic data more comparable on an etic dimension.

A variety of instruments are available for cross-cultural assessment. Some approaches, such as projective techniques, have been characterized as relativistic but have promise also in identifying universal patterns. Personality inventories have enjoyed rapidly increasing popularity across cultural boundaries, but the emphasis has been more on clinical prediction than on identification of cultural differences. Draguns correctly contends that some form of diversified measure for psychophysiological patterns of similarity and difference is needed in the assessment area.

Draguns concludes that although standardized self-report verbal instruments are the most popular assessment measures, they do not provide a systematic correction of misconceptions in matching culture and disorder. There is an imbalance of assessment measures that favor the etic conceptualization of disorder, emphasizing similarities and deemphasizing differences. More work is needed to develop projective techniques and especially physiological measures to counteract the dominance of an etic research strategy. Without a complementary balance of emic and etic variables, assessment data are likely to overemphasize disorder to the exclusion of mental health and prevent the diversification of measures.

Raymond Prince describes an exciting new area of physiological measures in his chapter on *exogenous* (outside) and *endogenous* (inside) factors. The body has endogenous healing factors for self-medication through a morphinelike system of endorphins that have a healing impact on pain and some illnesses. Healing, as Prince describes the process, involves both the endogenous and exogenous factors of the system. Research has demonstrated that endorphins, produced in hyperstress and hyperarousal states, can be stimulated by dreams and external stimuli such as films. Endogenous healing mechanisms might also include dissociated states, religious experiences, and even some forms of psychoses. Although the study of endorphins has great promise as a physiological resource for mental health, the data are far from conclusive and the experimental findings thus far tend to be tentative. However, the complementarity of endogenous and exogenous factors once again emphasizes the complexity of mental health across cultures.

In Chapter 4, Allen German describes the importance of universal factors in the systematic study of schizophrenia as a disorder across cultures. Extensive research by the World Health Organization has led the shift away from "belief-based" essentialism to operational scientific inquiry that rejects simplistic single-mechanism- or single-illness-type formulations. In the past, cross-cultural research has emphasized social and cultural distinctions with less emphasis on physical and biological factors.

German is critical of the "cross-cultural" perspective and prefers a comparative ecology perspective as more in keeping with the objectivity of basic research. We cannot yet suppose that schizophrenia is universally identifiable as an entity. Questionnaires have not yet been able to measure the complex variables of schizophrenia. It would appear that all cultures have some form of schizophrenia and that it may be benign, remitting, or malignant. These findings assume a fundamental and universal type of human response to some unknown pathology.

There are several conclusions possible from existing data on schizophrenia. First, reliable assessment is becoming possible across cultures. Second, schizophrenia is not the exclusive property of a specific society "type." Third, schizophrenia is described as morbid and pathological by both traditional healers and the general public. Fourth, traditional predictors of outcome are not reliable. Fifth, diagnosis is generally stable and consistent. More research is needed on the incidence, cultural problems, biological variables, and defining features of schizophrenia as a complex but universal example of mental illness.

In Chapter 5, Madeleine Leininger introduces the concept of "culturological assessment" to describe a comprehensive interview format that takes a broad view of the client's cultural context. In her guidelines, which she describes as the "Sunrise Model," she draws from her own experience as an anthropologist and as a nurse to describe a holistic perspective. The complexity of mediating between cultural conflicts and health care becomes apparent in Leininger's transcultural approach.

The final chapter on culture-general applications is by Harriet Lefley, on delivering mental health services across cultures. Lefley, a psychologist and faculty member of the University of Miami Department of Psychiatry, emphasizes several issues affecting the intercultural reliability and validity of existing models of health care. How can traditional healing be integrated with more global, universally accepted approaches? How can Western models of health care be implemented in culturally sensitive ways? How can existing healing systems be utilized most efficiently? What is a culturally sensitive service delivery system? What are the effects of cross-cultural research findings on the future of health care?

Modern mental health has been dominated by a pharmacological revolution toward treatment and a philosophical revolution toward community health care. Lefley describes the existing system as institutionalized racism resulting in differential treatment and outcome goals with massive avoidance behavior by professionals working with culturally different clients. An "open systems" conceptualization of mental health care is probably preferred, but institutionalization without community resources would be extremely problematic. An emphasis on American core values of independence and self-reliance has eroded community responsibility in health care. Alternative service delivery models have emphasized the family role, folk healing, and a community mental health rationale.

The significant issues described by Lefley include the following: (1) the need for a conceptual definition of mental health services, (2) service priorities and chronicity, (3) allocation of resources, (4) prevention, and (5) community participation. Like the other authors in Part I, Lefley advocates an integrated, wide-spectrum approach to mental health care with social, medical, environmental, ecological, and therapeutic approaches. Through this multimethod variety of approaches, including both culture-general and culture-specific perspectives, indigenous healing approaches can be integrated with Western systems in a more comprehensive perspective.

Part I brings to bear the viewpoints of two psychologists, a nurse-anthropologist, and two psychiatrists. In each case the direction of progress suggests an integration of emic and etic perspectives for mental health, toward a more comprehensive and necessarily

defn mhealth MENTAL HEALTH SERVICES

complex understanding of mental health services. Even in the study of schizophrenia, which has been one of the most promising universal patterns in the study of mental health, the culture-specific emic variable contributes to the "comparative ecology" of mental health.

CULTURE-SPECIFIC APPLICATIONS

Part II, on culture-specific applications, focuses on five different cultural settings by four anthropologists, three psychologists, and a medical doctor. In each cultural setting the authors emphasize the interrelationships that contribute to or detract from mental health.

Anthony Marsella and Howard Higginbotham, in their chapter on applying traditional Asian medicine explain why Western-oriented services have failed to take root in Asian countries. Omnibus healing centers have a potential for replacing Western-oriented hospitals while integrating Western methods with Asian healing systems. Such an omnibus service would need to grow out of an awareness of local traditions, an assessment of services for cultural accommodation, an increase in empirical data on patients, an incorporation of traditional healers, and the definition of mental health as harmonious relationships among physical, psychological, and spiritual concepts in a unified perspective.

Joseph Trimble, Spero Manson, Norman Dinges, and Beatrice Medicine describe the increased interest and literature on American Indians, even though most of the work is being done by non-Indians. There is a sense in which the Euro-American values violate traditional Indian cultural perspectives. The authors examine six basic tribal-specific concepts of disorder to demonstrate the variety of differences within the larger American Indian community. In each case, the Western definition of mental health—related to the biomedical balance or imbalance between mind and body—takes a "separateness" orientation inconsistent with Indian linguistic groups. Most Indian mental health has been described from within the Euro-American perspective in spite of this basic difference of value orientation.

The frequent errors of interpretation by non-Indians have resulted from reliance on a limited set of informants, unjustified generalization from specific cultural patterns, and failure to take the functional aspects of a phenomenon into account. There is need to focus on the context and indigenous theories of personhood to achieve or define successful psychosocial functions. Only those general patterns that can accommodate local values will provide meaningful mental health services.

In Chapter 9, Thomas Maretzki describes the realities of mental health service development in Indonesia. He takes the position that any matching of the indigenous and Western perspectives has to be decided by the Indonesians themselves and cannot be imposed by outside agencies. He suggests that there has been little feedback of value from findings and ideas generated by social scientists relating the basic research in culture and mental health to the needs of Indonesia. Maretzki emphasizes the importance of the ethnomedical model for future research in Indonesia and elsewhere in response to the "realities" of cultural complexity. These reality factors include cultural diversity, lack of a dominant traditional medical system, a legacy of mental health systems oriented toward severe disorders, and changes arising from the dynamic growth of an independent nation such as Indonesia. In Maretzki's view the narrowly focused Western system is yielding to a broader community mental health approach and more recently toward primary care by individual communities.

In Chapter 10, Erika Bourguignon provides another case-study perspective of belief, possession, and trance in Haiti. *Vodou* provides an example of African and Afro-American religion as a mental health resource that frequently contrasts with Western health care procedures. Although vodou began in the 1920s, it was not officially recognized until the 1960s. The altered state of consciousness brought about through vodou was classified as a form of hysteria. Possession trance plays an important role in Haitian folk healing, along with spirit possession, soul loss, and sudden fright as a part of the vodou perspective. The Haitian concepts of personality and health combine African, French, Catholic, and Caribbean perspectives in a unique combination that has now *become* an emic of vodou for Haitian culture.

In Chapter 11, Takeo Doi describes his own personal experience in relating his medical and psychological training in the United States to the more traditional Japanese setting. He begins with the premise that psychotherapies are rooted in their cultures of origin. Consequently, there is a need for sensitivity when clients and therapists are from different cultures. Finally, the tendency in modern times has been to adopt psychotherapies outside their cultures of origin. Doi's classic work on *amae* and the role of dependency has demonstrated that the dependency need is instrumental for interpersonal relationships. He describes the measure of dependency need through analogy to the children's games of hide-and-seek and peekaboo, based on patterns of familiarity and unfamiliarity in early infancy. In his search for a unified theory of psychotherapy, he has focused on interpersonal relationships as the key element. Non-Westeren therapies mingle the explorative and the supportive aspects, while in Western societies they are separated. The devination (diagnosis) and treatment (service) by a shaman takes place as a single event outside the Western setting.

The culture-specific applications continue the theme of complexity in understanding cultural aspects of mental health. Arguments for the use of indigenous healing methods emphasize their effectiveness in managing psychiatric disorder, the shortage and expense of Western psychiatric facilities, their high prestige in home cultures, and evidence that Western treatment modes tend to be culture bound (Prince, 1980). Both the outside Western (etic) and the inside indigenous (emic) provide valuable perspectives in a comprehensive mental health service. Where Western psychologies have emphasized the psyche or mind as a clinical target, non-Western cultures have more inclusively emphasized the interdependence of mind and matter, soul and body. Western therapies that are characterized by personal growth and self-exploration have, in some cases, led to increased adaptational difficulties as clients become more aware of and dissatisfied with their own context (Wohl, 1981). Seward (1970) argues that many traditional theories of psychothotherapy emphasize the individual as an isolated biosocial unit, without acknowledging the complex cultural effect on personality development. Western therapies teach individualistic self-scrutiny and critical analysis where the cause of neurotic and psychosomatic disorder is presumed to be embedded in the individual's basic personality. Lasch (1978) describes how the origins and maintenance of mental illness are perceived as rooted in the individual rather than in the social unit itself. Pande (1969) provided the classic satirical characterization of "exotic" Western perspectives where adulthood is the symbolic goal in which one attains values of self-reliance, power, achievement, responsibility, and sexual fulfillment independent of others.

The tendency has been to look for pathology in the client while overlooking the pathology of the surrounding environment (King, 1978; Sampson, 1977).

MEDIATORS OF
MENTAL HEALTH SERVICES

The therapist working in a culturally inclusive mode takes on the role of a mediator. Meadows (1968) discusses an early Greek notion of the therapist as mediating between the client and a superordinate world of powers and values. As mediator, the therapist role resembles Stonequist's (1937) "marginal" person, attempting to maintain a dual cultural identity. The therapist needs to develop skills of constant adaptation to new value configurations as a process rather than belonging to any one particular culture.

Weidman (1975), in working with culturally different clients, describes intermediaries as "culture brokers" attentive to the culturally inclusive loyalties of their clients and themselves. Miles (1976) has demonstrated how these "boundary spanning" activities can result in role ambiguity and role diffusion for the "integrator" or boundary role person who is expected to coordinate the conflicting demands of multiple membership. As mediators, the therapists may not have a complete understanding of the several cultures in which they work, but they can still link the cultures together based on inferences.

Truly "bicultural" individuals have the potential to function with cognitive flexibility and are creatively adaptive in either culture from which they draw their identities (Berry, 1975). The bicultural and bilingual mediator would understand the language patterns peculiar to a range of identities within each cultural community and would be acceptable as an "interpreter" by members of either community. The interpreter role needs to be well defined and accepted by both cultures to function effectively (MacKinnon & Michels, 1971).

Taft (1977) identifies a range of adaptive options for persons affiliated with more than one cultural reference group from encapsulation on the one extreme to the creation of a new third culture alternative at the other extreme. In any case, multicultural group membership is a normal and expected aspect of belonging to a complex society with contrasting values and attitudes. The ability to function competently and effectively in more than one cultural world is a necessary skill for the culturally inclusive therapist. Complexity provides a plurastic contrast to the "melting pot" analogy, where the primary goal would be to contribute toward a single culturally exclusive system. The "salad bowl" analogy may be more appropriate, where each element remains its individual identity while contributing to the whole.

There is evidence (LeVine & Campbell, 1972) that groups or individuals who perceive themselves to be quite similar are more likely to relate harmoniously. Members of the same subjective culture (Triandis, Vassiliou, Vassiliou, Tanaka, & Shanmugan, 1972) share a way of using concepts and value priorities in their interrelationships, while persons who differ in their ways of perceiving important elements of the subjective culture tend to dislike each other and are likely to have difficulties reaching agreements. The greater the differences, the greater the need for mediation.

The use of mediators in therapy is not a new idea. Bolman (1968) suggests that at least two therapists, one representing each culture, be used in cross-cultural therapy to provide a conceptual bridge between the counselor and client. Slack and Slack (1976) advocate bringing in a third resource person who has already coped effectively with the client's problem to interpret the advantages of counseling to the chemically dependent client. Mediators have been described in family therapy for treatment of pathogenic coalitions (Satir, 1964), with the therapist mediating judiciously to change pathogenic relating styles. Therapy resembles a series of negotiations in which all parties vie for control. Zuk (1971) describes this approach as a go-between process in which the therapist is a catalyst for conflict in a crisis situation, where all parties can have an active role. Barriers of language, class-bound values, and culture-bound goals weaken the therapist-client coalition to disrupt mental health services.

CONCLUSION

Draguns (1975) describes psychotherapy as a procedure that is sociocultural in its ends and interpersonal in its means. The literature on ethnography, ethnoscience, epidemiology, and cultural systems attacks what Kleinman (1978) calls a "discipline-bound compartmentalization" of medical research. The cultural context reveals the cognitive, behavioral, and institutional basis of it's structure, including the value and symbolic meanings underlying and determining that structure.

Increased knowledge and more sophisticated methodologies in the field of mental health reveal a complex relationship between specific cultures and the general descriptions of mental health therapies, services, and diagnoses across those cultural boundaries. Complexity provides an alternative to the "either/or" polarization of emic and etic categories by introducing the "both/and" complementarity perspective, where each event is viewed from *both* emic and etic viewpoints. Attempts to classify cultural phenomena exclusively in emic or etic categories have not been successful. Complementarity may provide an alternative perspective to accommodate the wealth of information now available about cultures and their interrelationships.

Five chapters emphasizing the culture-general perspective review the importance of including complex and comprehensive features of a culture to assess accurately the influence of mental health services. Both the exogenous and the endogenous factors are included in a comparative ecological relationship of interacting cultures. The appropriate delivery of mental health services assumes a broad and inclusive definition of culture by the outside provider of those services.

Five chapters emphasizing the culture-specific perspective review the application of Western perspectives of mental health on non-Western cultures. Each setting demonstrates the importance of etic categories in interpreting emic data within the context of an indigenous definition of health.

The chapters in this book describe a complex relationship between cultures and mental health services, therapies, and diagnoses being implemented in those cultures. The provider of mental health services will require both the general and the specific perspectives to interpret culturally appropriate mental health.

Each of the chapters emphasizes either a culture-general or a culture-specific perspective. The general chapters focus primarily on techniques, methods, or treatments going across cultures. The specific chapters focus primarily on specific populations describing the cultural context of mental health services. The concluding chapter synthesizes guidelines and observations that integrate both specific and general perspectives. While there are many techniques, methods, or treatments not included in this book, just as there are many additional populations not mentioned, the chapters will build on these selected examples to demonstrate our point. Both the general and specific perspectives are important.

REFERENCES

Andre, R. (1981). Multicultural research: Developing a participative methodology for cross-cultural psychology. *International Journal of Psychology, 16*, 249-256.

Atkinson, D., Morton, G., & Sue, D. W. (1979). *Counseling American minorities: A cross-cultural perspective.* Dubuque, IA: William C. Brown.

Bartunek, J. M., Gordon, J. R., & Weathersby, R. P. (1983). Developing "complicated" understanding in administrators. *Academy of Management Review, 8*(2), 273-284.

Berry, J. (1975). Ecology, cultural adaptation and psychological differentiation: Traditional patterning and acculturative stress. In R. Brislin, S. Bochner, & W. Lonner (Eds.), *Cross-cultural perspectives on learning* (pp. 207-231). New York: John Wiley.

Berry, J. (1980). Ecological analysis for cross-cultural psychology. In N. Warren (Ed.), *Studies in cross-cultural psychology* (Vol. 2). London: Academic.

Bohr, N. (1950). On the notion of causality and complementarity. *Science, 11*, 51-54.

Bolman, W. (1968). Cross-cultural psychotherapy. *American Journal of Psychiatry, 124*, 1237-1244.

Brislin, R. (1983). Cross-cultural research in psychology. *Annual Review of Psychology, 34*, 363-400.

Draguns, J. G. (1975). Resocialization into culture: The complexities of taking a world-wide view of psychotherapy. In R. Brislin, S. Bochner, & W. Lonner (Eds.), *Cross-cultural perspectives on learning.* New York: John Wiley.

Eiseman, J. (1978). Reconciling "incompatible" positions. *Journal of Applied Behavioral Science 14*, 133-150.

Favazza, A. F., & Oman, M. (1977). *Anthropological and cross-cultural themes in mental health: An annotated bibliography 1925-1974.* Columbia: University of Missouri Press.

Fowler, J. W. (1981). *Stages of faith.* New York: Harper & Row.

Gardner, C. S. (1972). Complexity training and prejudice reduction. *Journal of Applied Social Psychology, 2*, 325-342.

Gilligan, C. (1982). *In a different voice.* Cambridge, MA: Harvard University Press.

Harvey, O. J., Hunt, D. E., & Schroder, H. M. (1961). *Conceptual systems and personality organization.* New York: John Wiley.

Kegan, R. (1982). *The evolving self.* Cambridge, MA: Harvard University Press.

King, L. M. (1978). Social and cultural influences on psychotherapy. *Annual Review of Psychology, 29*, 405-433.

Kleinman, A. (1978). International health care planning from an ethno-medical perspective: Critique and recommendations for change. *Medical Anthropology, 2*(2), 71-96.

Kohlberg, L. (1969). Stage and sequence: The cognitive development approach to socialization. In D. Goslin (Ed.), *Handbook of socialization theory and research* (pp. 347-389). Chicago: Rand McNally.

Lasch, C. (1978). *The culture of narcissism.* New York: Norton.

LeVine, R., & Campbell, D. (1972). *Ethnocentrism: Theories of conflict, ethnic attitudes and group behavior.* New York: John Wiley.

Lonner, W. (1980). The search for psychological universals. In H. Triandis & W. Lambert (Eds.), *Handbook of cross-cultural psychology* (Vol. 1). Boston: Allyn & Bacon.

Lovinger, J. (1976). *Ego development.* San Francisco: Jossey-Bass.

MacKinnon, R. A., & Michels, R. (1971). *The psychiatric interview in clinical practice.* Philadelphia: W. B. Saunders.

Marsella, A. J. (1980). Depressive experience and disorder across cultures. In H. C. Triandis & J. G. Draguns (Eds.), *Handbook of cross-cultural psychology: Vol. 2. Methodology.* Boston: Allyn & Bacon.

Marsella, A. J., & Petersen, P. (Eds.). (1981). *Cross-cultural counseling and psychotherapy.* Elmsford, NY: Pergamon.

Marsella, A. J., & White, G. M. (Eds.). (1982). *Cultural conceptions of mental health and therapy.* Dordrecht: D. Reidel.

Meadows, P. (1968). The cure of souls and the winds of change. *Psychoanalytic Review, 44,* 491-504.

Miles, R. H. (1976). Role requirements as sources of organizational stress. *Journal of Applied Psychology, 61,* 172-179.

Pande, S. K. (1969). The mystique of Western psychotherapy: An Eastern interpretation. *Journal of Nervous and Mental Disorders, 146,* 425-432.

Pedersen, P., Draguns, J., Lonner, W., & Trimble, J. (1981). (Eds.). *Counseling across cultures.* Honolulu: University Press of Hawaii.

Perry, W. G. (1970). *Forms of intellectual and ethical development in the college years: A scheme.* New York: Holt, Rinehart & Winston.

Pike, R. (1966). *Language in relation to a united theory of the structure of human behavior.* The Hague: Mouton.

Prince, R. (1980). Variations in psychotherapeutic procedures. In H. C. Triandis & J. G. Draguns (Eds.), *Handbook of cross-cultural psychology: Vol. 6. Psychopathology.* Boston: Allyn & Bacon.

Sampson, E. (1977). Psychology and the American ideal. *Journal of Personality and Social Psychology, 11,* 767-782.

Satir, V. (1964). *Conjoint family therapy.* Palo Alto, CA: Science and Behavior Books.

Schroder, H., Driver, M., & Streufert, S. (1967). *Human information processing.* New York: Holt, Rinehart & Winston.

Seward, G. (1970). *Clinical studies in cultural conflict.* New York: Ronald.

Slack, C. W., & Slack, E. N. (1976, February). It takes three to break a habit. *Psychology Today,* pp. 46-50.

Stonequist, F. U. (1937). *The marginal man: A study in personality and culture conflict.* New York: Russell & Russell.

Taft, R. (1977). Coping with unfamiliar environments. In N. Warren (Ed.), *Studies of cross-cultural psychology* (Vol. 1). London: Academic.

Triandis, H. C. (1977). *Interpersonal behavior.* Monterey, CA: Brooks/Cole.

Triandis, H. C., Vassiliou, V., Vassiliou, G., Tanaka, Y., & Shanmugan, A. V. (1972). *The analysis of subjective culture.* New York: John Wiley.

Trimble, J. E., Lonner, W. J., & Boucher, J. D. (1983). *Stalking the wily emic: Alternatives to cross-cultural measurement.* Bellingham: Western Washington University.

Weidman, H. (1975). Concepts as strategies for change. *Psychiatric Annals, 5,* 312-314.

Wohl, J. (1981). Can we export Western psychotherapy to non-Western cultures? In P. Pedersen, J. Draguns, W. Lonner, & J. Trimble (Eds.), *Counseling across cultures* (rev. ed.). Honolulu: University Press of Hawaii.

Zuk, G. (1971). *Family therapy: A triadic based approach.* New York: Behavioral Publications.

I: Culture-General Applications

2

ASSESSING MENTAL HEALTH
AND DISORDER ACROSS
CULTURES

JURIS G. DRAGUNS

The assessment of mental health and disorder in several cultures poses a serious methodological challenge to behavioral sciences and mental health professions. The problems of assessing a person's state of psychological well-being or disorder objectively, reliably, and validly in a monocultural setting are not yet fully resolved. These problems are augmented as psychological disturbance at two or more culturally distinct sites is being assessed. In particular, the problem of how to differentiate behavior that is disturbed and pathological from behavior that is culturally characteristic must be faced. A culturally naive observer with a universalistic conception of psychopathology runs the risk of confounding culturally distinctive behavior with psychopathological manifestations on the basis of surface similarities of behavior patterns in a different culture to psychiatric symptomatology at the observer's home base. Take the example of hallucinations, thoroughly analyzed in the cross-cultural context by Al-Issa (1977, 1978). This behavior is considered symptomatic of psychosis in the West and, in a wide range of circumstances, in a great many non-Western cultures as well. However, Al-Issa (1977, 1978) notes, there are noteworthy exceptions where the experience of hallucinations in a particular cultural context may be not only tolerated, but indeed prescribed. Individuals who exhibit such experiences are not only exempted from ostracism and other forms of social rejection and degradation—indeed, the possession of the gift to communicate with the spirits may be an indispensable prerequisite to the performance of a number of culturally prized tasks and roles (see Boyer, Klopfer, Brawer, & Kawai, 1964; Fabrega & Silver, 1973; Dinges, Trimble, Manson, & Pasquale, 1981). It is the loss of this gift that would bring about impairment of social status and other frustrations.

Confounding of culture with psychopathology is then one of the obstacles that must be overcome in developing a mode of culturally sensitive and yet realistic assessment. The other problem is confounding psychopathology with deviance. Psychopathology is the more narrow subcategory within the broader class of social deviance. Only "residual" deviance, not readily explained by recourse to information generally available within a culture, is psychopathological (Scheff, 1966). Confounding of social deviance with psychopathology can and does occur even on home grounds, in culturally uniform settings. The dangers of such occurrence, however, are magnified when an unfamiliar culture is faced in which behavior deviating from, or violating, its norms occurs. A person familiar with both culture and psychopathology will in the optimal case be able to make the subtle distinction between sensible infringement of cultural rules and idiosyncratic assault upon cultural barriers. Finally, as pointed out elsewhere (Draguns, 1973), in the assessment of psychopathology and its comparison across cultural lines, there is the danger of confounding the effects of the observer, the (treatment or institutional) setting, and the community with those of culture on the one hand and disorder on the other.

Against the background of these possible pitfalls, my task is to review and evaluate the current state of assessment of psychological disorder and health across cultures, with an emphasis upon advances in instrumentation and methodology, unsolved problems and unfinished tasks, and prospects and need for the future. In so doing, I will lean and rely upon my earlier writings on this subject (Draguns, 1977a, 1982) and contributions of other authors who have addressed themselves to the problems of this field (Marsella, 1978, 1979; Murphy, 1969).

THE DEVELOPMENT OF
SYMPTOM-BASED MEASURES

By comparison with the early, premethodological stages of cross-cultural study of psychological disturbance, great progress has been made in objectifying and operationalizing the tasks of the psychiatric observer, assessor, or diagnostician. By contrast to arriving at a diagnostic categorization by means of operations unspecified, modern psychiatric researchers have at their command an array of instruments that enable them to anchor, check, and compare their judgments.

The development of this instrumentation has, as Kendell (1973) has pointed out, rendered obsolete the often-repeated and widely quoted conclusion on the low reliability of psychiatric diagnosis (see Spitzer & Fleiss, 1974). The reliability of diagnostic assignment increases under two kinds of circumstances: (1) when the amount of information to be processed in arriving at a diagnostic decision is severely and artifically limited, for example, by restricting the prediagnostic data collection to five minutes and specifying what information to collect; and (2) when the process and product of psychiatric assessment is standardized in the form of a detailed interview schedule, complete with instructions for the process of information gathering and symptom rating and recording. The former development is not directly germane to the increase of reliability in gathering psychological data across culture lines. While it may substantially decrease the proportion of variable errors, it does nothing to eliminate consensually shared or culturally constant ones. The latter approach has been exceedingly influential in getting systematic cross-cultural observation of abnormal behavior off the ground. The development of such standardized tools of assessment has been a process of mutual influence by the parent discipline of objective descriptive psychopathology and the specialized field of cross-cultural psychiatric assessment. Cross-cultural investigators of abnormal behavior have not simply borrowed and applied the methodology of objective, quantified, and standardized psychiatric observation, recording, and inference to the problem of psychiatric assessment in to or more cultures. In the case of two of the more prominent tools of such appraisal, Present Status Schedule (PSS), developed by Spitzer, Endicott, Fleiss, and Cohen (1970), and Present Status Examination (PSE), by Wing (Wing, Cooper, & Sartorius, 1974), the major arena of their application, revision, and refinement has been through cross-cultural research, notably the U.S.-U.K. study (Cooper et al., 1972) and the continuing World Health Organization (1973, 1979) study of schizophrenia. Similarly, the Katz Adjustment Scale (Katz, Sanborn, Lowery, & Ching, 1978) has seen one of its most thorough and searching applications in the multiethnic setting of Hawaii, while the Inpatient Multidimensional Psychiatric Scale, developed by Lorr (1966), has been applied in a series of multicultural factorial studies (Lorr & Klett, 1968, 1969a,

1969b). Similarly, the Brief Psychiatric Rating Scale developed by Overall and Gorham (1962) served as the principal tool in a collaborative multinational project concerned with the empirical bases of severeal national diagnostic systems (Engelsmann et al., 1971).

The above instruments were designed for the study of the entire range of psychopathology. Over a more limited span of psychopathological experiences, such instruments as those developed by Hamilton (1967) and Zung (1969) have been often adopted for use beyond their cultural boundaries; the Comprehensive Depressive Symptom Checklist (Marsella & Sanborn, 1973) has been specifically designed for use in multicultural settings. Similarly, at least three of the currently prominent paper-and-pencil measures of anxiety, the Spielberger State-Trait Anxiety Inventory (Spielberger & Diaz Guerrero, 1976), the IPAI Anxiety Scale (Cattell & Scheier, 1961), and the S-R Inventory of General Trait Anxiousness (Endler & Magnusson, 1976), have been used extensively in cross-cultural research. The Langner (1962) stress inventory has been widely investigated in several cultural settings and is especially frequently used in studies of migrated or displaced populations (for example, see Lasry, 1975, 1977). In fact, without much exaggeration, one can conclude that cross-cultural investigators of psychopathology are only second to psychopharmacological investigators in their reliance upon standardized interview schedules, symptom checklists, and systematic measures of negative affect states (Norton, 1967; Phillips & Draguns, 1971; Villeneuve, 1970; Wittenborn, 1972; Zubin, 1967).

The reason for this marriage of convenience between the developers of paper-and-pencil tools of psychiatric assessment and the investigators of the relationship of psychopathology in several cultures is the particularly strong need for objectification and standardization, related to the danger of the several kinds of confounding, alluded to earlier in this chapter. There is no doubt that these kinds of instruments have demonstrated their usefulness in a number of important projects. Thus the reliance upon a combination of PSE and PSS enabled the researchers in the U.S.-U.K. project to assign the source of the dramatic difference between the two countries of depression and schizophrenia to diagnosticians of the two countries, rather than to the patients. Whether this difference is truly artifactual—that is, the result of haphazardly divergent patterns of diagnostic practice in these two English-speaking countries—or whether it represents true differences in the thresholds for depression and schizophrenia, respectively, in these two cultures remains at this point unclear, but at least the most apparent possibility, that of a true difference in incidence, has been decisively and conclusively excluded.

In the two reports emanating from the World Health Organization study of schizophrenia (World Health Organization, 1973, 1979), the existence of a uniform "core group" of schizophrenics at the nine research centers around the world has been documented and meaningful differences in the course of illness, especially in developing versus developed countries included in this multicultural comparison, have been recorded. Cross-cultural differences in the self-reported levels of depressed affect have been recorded (Zung, 1969, 1972) and parallels drawn with analogous measures in psychiatric populations and suicide rates in the same countries. Use of these kinds of instruments has enabled research psychiatrists and clinical psychologists to compare the characteristics of very different patient populations. Moreover, the development of these tools and their adaptation for use across cultural and linguistic barriers has made possible the extension of these variables beyond the range found in any one culture. Thus the potential has been created for making the theory of psychopathology more precise by identifying cultures in which people seem to behave out of line with predictions based on theoretical models that have originated in a specific country, most typically the United States. For example, epidemiological research in Sweden (Leighton et al., 1971) has demonstrated that the association between low socioeconomic status and incidence of psychiatric disturbance, previously observed in the United States and Canada and present on a worldwide basis in reviews of epidemiological research by Dohrenwend and Dohrenwend (1974), does not hold in that country. More generally, the World Health Organization (1979) team of collaborating investigators has produced evidence on the surprising susceptibility of high-status individuals among the patient population of the research treatment centers in developing countries to a chronic course of the disorder, reversing the relationship observed and documented in the West. Another finding from the same research project pertains to a more benign source of schizophrenia in developing rather than developed countries (Cooper & Sartorius, 1977), a finding that extends and corroborates earlier reports by Murphy and Raman (1971), Raman and Murphy (1972), Waxler (1979), and others.

None of these increases in our knowledge would have been possible or at least likely were it not for the development and application of these measures. Parallel to this advance in methodology, there has been a corresponding increase in the sophistication of the technology of translation of verbal measures. Admittedly, most of these developments (Brislin, 1970, 1976; Prince & Mombour, 1967; Sechrest, Fay, & Zaidi, 1972; Wagatsuma, 1977) have occurred outside of the field of cross-cultural study of abnormal behavior, but they have been found applicable to a wide range of instruments of psychiatric interest. As recently as two decades ago, paper-and-pencil scales were translated without the benefit of specific safeguards: back-translation, reconciling discrepancies in conference, checking on linguistic and social appropriateness with the help of key informants, and pretesting the translation on a sample of bilingual individuals. All of these precautions are now widely, if not universally adopted.

More problematic and difficult to attain are the recommendations by Brislin (1976) for writing generically translatable prose that puts a premium on grammatical and semantic simplicity, redundancy, and clarity of the original. The problem is that as of this date, few instruments are designed explicitly for use in translation. Moreover, especially in the case of investigation of subtle and complex experiences and states, a condition quite often encountered in research on psychopathology, the question remains open whether the purpose of the inquiry can be attained while abiding by all of Brislin's (1976) recommendations. The answer to this question is, of course, empirical and awaits the determination of the actual limits within which this procedure can be applied. So far, I have not encountered any accounts in the research literature on the actual problems in reconciling translatability and complexity of content, but psychopathology is a likely area in which such problem may occur.

Another problem characteristic of, although not unique to, cross-cultural psychopathology pertains to the difficulty in translating terms that describe subjective emotional states. Experience demonstrates that translations of these terms often diverge in terms of their intensity, commonality, and range of usage even when their denotative dictionary meaning is the same. Wagatsuma (1977) deserves the credit for addressing this problem directly. Even in languages as close in structure and vocabulary as English, French, and German, there are problems of diverging connotations even in the face of constant denotative meaning. For example *dickkopfig* is the equivalent of "hardheaded," but with a definite negative valence, as in the English word "pigheaded," but not quite as strongly; *"rigoureux"* is about right in valence for "hardheaded," but is limited to a more narrow range of usage, mostly concerned with cognitive and intellectual matters. The examples could be extended, and indeed are in Wagatsuma's (1977, p. 143) article. They collectively point to the difficulty, perhaps near impossibility, of coming up with *le mot juste* in translation. A partial remedy is contained in one of Brislin's (1976) recommendations: Embed the word in context, do not use it in isolation. From this point of view, adjective checklists would appear to be among the most difficult instruments to translate; my limited experience tends to corroborate this conclusion.

A special translation problem is encountered in multicultural investigations, such as the World Health Organization (1973, 1979) studies. In practice, translations into several project languages are made from English. This, however, opens the possibility of uncontrolled slippage of the several translations in different directions. The ideal solution would be translation from and to all of the project languages. In practical terms, the task of finding translators who are fluent in, for example, Danish and Yoruba, or Hindi and Czech, may prove to be impossible. Still, at least some lateral translations would be better than none; absence of differences btween, say, Czech and Russian, and Danish and Spanish versions might suggest that similar errors are at least unlikely in the remaining translations.

Translation, however, is not the only kind of adaptation that the use of paper-and-pencil instruments across culture lines may require. Two important characteristics to be considered are the content and the format of the measure. Both may vary in cultural relevance and appropriateness. On the former point, the further the investigator moves from his or her home base culturally, not necessarily geographically, the greater the problem with the fit of the content of the items. "I would rather advance my personal welfare than venerate the spirits of my ancestors"—an actual item from a personality scale in Japan—would strike most American respondents as odd and, in any case, irrelevant: It is a choice they do not expect to encounter in their lives and one on which they have no ready-made opinion. Conversely, the item on the MMPI, "I wish I were not so shy," is about as meaningful in Japan as the statement "I wish I were not so sociable" is in the United States. Certainly, in both cases, the endorsements of the items would be quite lopsided in the direction of behavior that in their respective countries is positively valued: gregariousness in the United States and decorous social reticence in

Japan. Going even further afield, the French research team of Zeldine et al. (1975) found that in Senegal as many as one-third of all the items of the Hamilton Depression Scale had to be discarded as being irrelevant to the African experience of depression. Conversely, several new items were added to reflect the culturally characteristic and locally prevalent complaints and expressions of depression. In a similar fashion, Durojaiye (1975) in Uganda made use of local informants in order to include characteristic modes of experiencing anxiety in a scale he was constructing for use with Ugandan high school students. These kinds of changes, through subtraction or addition, raise the question of the cross-cultural equivalence of the final product. They also introduce the issue, to be discussed at greater length later, of the differential pull toward cross-cultural equivalence and cultural sensitivity (see Draguns, 1982).

On a more general plane, the construction of paper-and-pencil tools of assessment has to contend with culturally mediated response styles. To answer affirmatively in several Far Eastern countries is a sign of politeness; to say no is to be rude. Even though most Far Eastern respondents are aware of the fact that this requirement does not extend to paper-and-pencil scale impersonally administered, the pull of lifelong training in polite acquiescence may be too strong and may result in yes or "agree" answers on a number of ambiguous or complex items. That such a tendency exists has been corroborated empirically in a study of Korean and American subjects by Chun, Campbell, and Yoo (1974). To put this finding in perspective, it has been established that, within a culture, a response set determines a detectable, but not major, share of the variance (Block, 1965; Rorer, 1965). There are no grounds for believing that these response styles assume greater importance cross-culturally. Nevertheless, they may be there and may exercise a noticeable pull in the direction of a particular kind of responding.

Finally, on the most general plane, the questionnaire format of self-disclosure is very likely subject to cross-cultural differences. As Boesch (1971) has pointed out, the ability to reveal one's own subjective state is a human universal, but the inclination to do so is culturally mediated. American investigators, coming from probably the most test-oriented culture in the world, often naively or unthinkingly assume that other cultures are equally "test wise" and prepared to submit to the standardized verbal limited-option format. The extent to which cultures vary in this characteristics has never been determined systematically or objectively. Casual observation suggests, however, that there is a great deal of cultural variation along this dimension. Quite possibly, the anxiety and the resistance that accompany the administration of self-report inventories may be the function of the novelty or surprise value of the administration of these instruments. Other cultural characteristics, such as prescribing self-disclosure only in specific and ritualized situations, may also come into play and may considerably complicate the administration of paper-and-pencil instruments of assessment and the response to them.

The foregoing considerations chiefly apply to the measures that are administered to psychiatric patients directly. The use of a psychiatrist, or other mental health professional, as a recorder of information by means of a standardized scale removes many of the cultural complications anticipated in the preceding sections of this chapter. But two different kinds of complications ensue. One of them is the reaction to the psychiatric interviewer and to the content of his or her questions, which may be culturally variable. The other factor is the information-processing style of the psychiatrist, a characteristic on which psychiatrists intraculturally have been found to vary (Gauron & Dickinson, 1966). Whether or not they so vary across cultures is a question on which we lack data.

The development of objective standardized measures that permit the reliable recording of symptoms and automatic derivation of diagnosis, such as from P.S.E. through the CATEGO procedure (Wing, Cooper, & Sartorius, 1974), is a great advance in the methodology of cross-cultural assessment of abnormal behavior. The bulk of research on psychopathology across cultures in the past decade has been done using this approach, characterized by the objective collection of symptom data. In the process, certain imbalances in the study of psychological disturbance in relation to culture have become apparent and need to be articulated.

ETIC BIAS AND HOW TO CORRECT IT

The kind of research so far described represents an *etic* strategy *par excellence*. The assumptions on which this approach rests is that cross-cultural differences are quantitative rather than qualitative and, on a less explicit level, that pan-cultural similarities in abnormal behavior by far outweigh cross-cultural differences. Finifter (1977)

has identified two implicit aims of cross-cultural research: universalist, geared toward demonstrating cross-cultural constancies; and
specifist, designed to highlight and articulate cross-cultural differences. A third type, according to Finifter (1977), is agnostic, which
provides an equal chance for the emergence of both differences and
similarities. In the cross-cultural study of abnormal behavior, by
comparison with a number of other areas of cross-cultural psychology, the universalist approach has been predominant. The assumption
has been that human psychopathology is basically universal,
although subsidiary differences, the local color of psychological
disturbance, have been granted.

   Along somewhat similar lines, several observers and evaluators of
cross-cultural psychiatric research (Draguns, 1977a, 1982; Marsella,
1978, 1979; Kleinman, 1977) are in agreement in concluding that the
emic approach in the systematic study of abnormal behavior has so
far not been given a fair chance. Exceptions to the pronouncedly etic
slant of most of the research on abnormal behavior across cultures are
for the most part in the form of descriptive accounts of culture-
specific syndromes (for example, see Murphy, 1972a; Tan & Carr,
1977; Yap, 1974), supplemented, in the case of some of the more
recent and innovative reports, by quantitative data from a variety of
prespectives. Tanaka-Matsumi (1979) has had the original idea of
presenting a number of case histories of *taijin-kyofusho*, the
Japanese version of social phobia (recognized of late in DSM III), to
American psychiatrists for diagnosis, thereby blending two cultural
systems and two modes of analysis in elucidating the nature of this
much-discussed syndrome. Epidemiological studies of culture-
specific syndromes are possible and have, on occasion, been
attempted, although Fabrega (1974) sees a conflict in confounding
two conceptions of psychopathology, folk and epidemiological.

   Marsella (1978) has probably gone furthest in proposing a
complete strategy of cross-cultural epidemiological investigation
resting on an emic foundation of case finding. Speaking specifically of
the epidemiology of depression, Marsella suggests a four-step
sequence. Frist, an emic determination of disorder categories in
different cultures uses the methods of ethnoscience, that is, to capture
and articulate the implicit taxonomy of these kinds of phenomena in
the cultural milieu in which they occur. Second, there is the establishment of symptom frequency, intensity, and duration baselines.
Monocultural research by Cohen (1967) and culturally oriented
studies by Marsella, Tanaka-Matsumi, and Sanborn (1974) demon-

strate that the relationship of these three parameters of symptomatology is complex, although it is not random. Third, once the units of disturbance have been emically determined and quantified in relation to their three basic characteristics, objective symptom patterns can be established by means of multivariate techniques of data analysis. Finally, comparative studies can be implemented using similar methodologies with culturally relevant definitions of disorder. This research strategy, which, as yet, has not been fully implemented, proceeds then from emic identification through quantification to etic comparison and provides a possible avenue of making emic data etically comparable.

STUDIES OF SUBJECTIVE EXPERIENCE, PHENOMENOLOGY, AND PSYCHODYNAMICS

Another slant that is detectable in the currently prominent objective symptom-based research strategy favors observable and reportable psychological reactions over subjective experience and phenomenology. Both monocultural studies, for the most part European (Minkowski, 1966; Tellenbach, 1976), and culturally oriented observations and comparisons (Kimura, 1965, 1967, 1972; Tellenbach, 1972) suggest that phenomenology of psychopathological experience is a rich source of important data. In reference to culture, it ties together a number of seemingly random and unrelated surface manifestations of the disorder. On the plane of explicitly designed systematic research, these kinds of subjective variables have rarely been explored. Tanaka-Matsumi and Marsella (1976) have explored the phenomenology of depressive experience as a function of culture and language by means of the word-association technique. Another unpublished article by the same research team has explored the semantic-differential ratings of depression-related stimuli in culturally and linguistically different groups (Tanaka-Matsumi & Marsella, 1977). Remarkably, a prominent research approach within the domain of cross-cultural social and personality psychology has, so far, not been used explicitly in the study of abnormal individuals. Reference here is to the cluster of measures employed in the study of the subjective culture by Triandis and others (Triandis, 1972, 1977). Vassiliou and Vassiliou (1974) of Greece have pointed out the problems that arise in the clinical setting when the therapists and the patients lack a shared subjective culture or, within a more conventional terminology, a common world view (also see Torrey, 1972; Stewart, 1981; Wohl, 1981). These illustrative case studies, however, are no substitute for the systematic application of the subjective culture measures to clinical and normal samples in two or more cultures.

Another way of both looking beneath the surface and correcting the etic-emic imbalance in psychopathological research is exemplified by the work of Doi (1973) on culturally distinctive psychodynamics, exemplified by the Japanese pattern of seeking lifelong dependent gratification, or *amae*. This work has led to the tentative development of paper-and-pencil scales designed to measure this characteristic. Other approaches for the study of amae can be envisaged, such as thematic, that could be directly based on themes and illustrations of Doi's writings.

While culturally characteristic psychodynamics have rarely been described, cultural variations and peculiarities in motivational forces may constitute a fertile field of investigation, both in their own right and in relation to cultural variations in psychopathology. A greater attention to such forces may be another way of redressing the emic-etic balance in our understanding of psychopathology in relation to culture.

PROJECTIVE TECHNIQUES AND THEIR ROLE IN CROSS-CULTURAL RESEARCH

A major approach to this end is available in the form of projective techniques. The literature on projective tests used in various cultures is voluminous and has experienced a number of ups and down over several decades. From the privileged and unique position as the putative key to the real personality structure and dynamics characteristically prevalent within a culture, the projective techniques shrank to the status of a distinctly minor and subsidiary approach in the study of cultural differences in personality. Lindzey's (1961) critical book-length treatment of the legitimate uses and the prevalent misuses of projective techniques stands as a watershed between the rise and decline of projective techniques in cultural psychology. Lindzey's (1961) criticisms are well known and scarcely need to be recapitulated here. What Lindzey did was to apply the then-current standards of personality research to what had been a field characterized by naturalistic, qualitative, and impressionistic approaches. Specifically, Lindzey objected to (a) use of central tendencies to describe the "typical" or "prevailing" personality structure on the basis of test data, while ignoring the degree of their variability within the group; (b) the nonrandom and often unspecified selection of subjects in the available reports on test results within the culture; (c) lack of systematic integration of projective test data with other available sources of information; (d) reliance upon subjective and haphazard impressions in the absence of such integration; (e) the neglect of possible examiner and situational influences as sources of alternative explanations of results obtained; (f) mechanistic use of rules of scoring and interpretation originating in Europe or North America and their unmodified application to other cultures; and (g) contamination of interpretation of test data by other sources of data.

As an alternative to these misuses of projective techniques, Lindzey advocated a culture-centered or emic approach based upon the revalidation of these techniques in each culture in which they were to be applied. Lindzey's criticisms are consonant with the views of Spain (1972), another critic of projective techniques. Collectively, these critical and analyses coincided with the decline of interest in culture and personality as a topic of research and conceptualization (Draguns, 1979a, 1979b, 1979c; Tapp, 1981). The culturally relativistic view of projective techniques came to be the conventional wisdom and was rarely called into question.

Two formulations, one conceptual and the other empirical, have failed to fit into this consensus. On the theoretical plane, DeVos (1965, 1976) has been a minority of one in upholding the universalistic view of projective techniques, especially the Rorschach. He sharply distinguishes adjustment and adaptation, the former indicative of progression through a universal series of maturational stages, the latter culturally available roles. Appropriate and realistic use of projective techniques requires that these two processes be kept apart and separately evaluated. A person may be mature, yet poorly adapted to cultural reality. In such a case, the tests would indicate a universally valid pattern of high psychological development and secondary signs of anxiety, frustration, or aggression associated with the conflict between the person and his or her milieu. As DeVos (1976, p. 298) says, "Psychological testing can be used cross-culturally. It can help us gain a glimpse into the personality structure of particular individuals and by so doing it helps sort out essential differences between observable role behavior and underlying personality." Elsewhere, he says, "Contrary to such opinions, I have found test materials with which I have become familiar to be generally valid and capable of being analyzed as is such material obtained from Americans" (DeVos, 1976, p. 288).

The other body of data that might stimulate the reexamination of the pronouncedly relativistic view of projective techniques has come from large-scale cross-cultural research with the new, psychometrically streamlined inkblot test, the Holtzman Inkblot Technique (HIT; Holtzman, 1980). Two findings have emerged from these uses of the HIT in several cultures: (1) The factorial structure of the HIT has proved to be remarkably constant in a number of very different cultural settings (Holtzman, 1980); (2) computerized interpretations of HIT findings have been shown to be valid in light of external criteria cross cultural boundaries (Gorham, 1970), These findings suggest that it may not in all cases be necessary to start from scratch when applying projective techniques in a new and different cultural milieu.

As far as the use of projective techniques as tools of cross-cultural assessment is concerned, it is not that they have been tried and rejected. Rather, they have never been put to this use seriously and systematically. Holtzman's (1980) recent and thorough review of cross-culturally use of projective techniques thoroughly documents and corroborates this assertion. To elaborate, the projective techniques have a rich and checkered history of being used as tools for the determination of "cultural personality" and modal personality structure. In some of this work, metaphors from diagnostic taxonomy have been used, sometimes loosely. This, however, is quite different from investigating psychopathology within and across a variety of cultures and using psychologically disturbed individuals to that end. This task has been only rarely and atypically undertaken and the degree of cross-cultural constancy, if any, of signs of psychopathology has been neither refuted nor established. DeVos (1965, 1976) cites only a limited number of studies that bear upon the alleged universality of indicators of psychosocial maturity in the Rorschach test. In the recent cultural literature, the work of Scheper-Hughes (1979) in western Ireland stands out for the intensive utilization of the TAT with both clinical (that is, psychiatrically hospitalized) and normal (without a history of psychological complaints or treatment for them) samples. However, the samples were small and no formal tests of statistical significance were applied. While Scheper-Hughes is quite impressed with the differences in need structure in her clinical and normal groups of subjects, these differences—converted from small raw differences into more impressive percentages—are not convincing.

On the basis of the present state of evidence, there is nothing to suggest that projective techniques—inkblots, thematic picture drawings, and others—could serve as cross-culturally constant and valid criteria of psychopathology. They could, however, be used as additional tools of appraisal, to provide information on perception and structuring of the external world and, especially, of the ambiguous portions thereof in addition to the information obtained in the course of more direct interchange between the examinee and the examiner. In this fashion, they would supplement, although they need not replace, the interview-based findings on present status, symptomatology, past history, and demographic data. Other as yet neglected sources of information pertain to data from the experimental laboratory.

PERSONALITY INVENTORIES: ADAPTATION FOR SENSITIVITY OR COMPARABILITY

While the use of projective techniques across cultures has declined, the application of personality inventories beyond cultural, linguistic, and national boundaries has experienced a marked recrudescence. This has been especially true of the MMPI (Butcher & Pancheri, 1975; Butcher & Clarke, 1978), which is well on the way to becoming a worldwide tool, used on all continents and translated into a score of languages. This effort, however, is principally aimed at the adaptation of the original Minnesota-based test for maximally effective intracultural use at its various new locales. The implementation of this objective involves, of necessity, the adaptation of wording and content. The result of such as undertaking is a new, if overlapping, test that is designed to perform optimally in intracultural use, but is ill fitted for cross-cultural comparisons with its original or with the versions of the test in other countries and languages. On an only slightly smaller scale, the same developments have been traversed by the State-Trait Anxiety Inventory (Spielberger & Diaz Guerrero, 1976). Sechrest et al. (1972) refer to the paradox of equivalence. As Sharma (1977, p. 170) explains it:

This paradox is that if one demands that a form of a test yield comparable results in two cultures in order to demonstrate equivalence, then the more equivalent the two forms become the less probability of finding cultural differences. On the other hand, if one looks predominantly for cultural differences and ignores the problem of equivalence, the greater the probability of cultural differences.

In essence, the adaptations of paper-and-pencil inventories across cultures capitalize on the former objective over the latter and, as a result, are a lot more useful for clinical use across cultures that they are for comparisons across cultures.

OTHER RESEARCH APPROACHES: EXPERIMENTAL, PHYSIOLOGICAL

If projective tests have but rarely been used in establishing differences between normal and disturbed groups in several cultures, the implementation of experimental studies of psychopathology with the cultural variable explicitly included is virtually nonexistent. Yet experimental research on psychopathology has been conducted in several cultures. It is unfortunate that the several reviews of such studies (for example, Rabin, Doneson, & Jentons, 1979) almost exclusively concentrate on American and English-language research reports. Conceivably, a more international survey might have uncovered some differences in findings of such studies, but as yet nobody has undertaken this kind of task. In its absence, we are faced with a potential avenue of cross-cultural comparison of abnormal behavior and of differences between normal and abnormal individuals.

The same considerations apply to the use of psychophysiological and physiological indicators. As far as I know, there have not as yet been any international or cross-cultural studies that have probed functioning "below the skin." That this would be fruitful area to explore is suggested by the observations of Murphy (1972b) and others that the response to psychoactive drugs may be to a limited extent culturally mediated. The point of departure for this work was the observation by Murphy that the dosages of psychoactive drugs recommended in the West European psychopharmaceutical literature were considerably lower than those prescribed in North America (see Joyce, 1980). In reference to the controversy surrounding the alleged universality of depressive phenomena and states (see Marsella, 1980), it would be interesting to establish the identity or difference of catecholamine levels in the floridly depressed guilt-ridden Westerners and West Africans demonstrating but a limited picture of vital signs of depression (Olatowura, 1973; Diop, 1967). The case for universalists would be much stronger if, in both settings, depression proved to be biologically identical. Again, in the absence of such work, one is left with the option of scrutinizing the available monocultural reports on the psychobiology of depressive states for clues to any differences that may eventually be demonstrated to be cultural.

In a more general way, the direction to be recommended is a multimethod approach that eschews reliance upon a single approach or a specific source of data. The pioneering studies by Opler and Singer (1959), on the differentiating features of schizophrenia in young Irish American and Italian American men, were based on a multiplicity of methods from observations of overt behavior to patterns of responses to projective tests. Somehow, this praiseworthy feature of this early study failed to be emulated while advances in the field came to be focused upon improvements of observational and recording methodology. Yet the call by Murphy (1969) for diversification as a basic research strategy continues to be as valid today as when it was first made. Two basic goals are attained through diversification: (1) Intraindividual variation across methods and perspectives provides glimpses into the complexity and variety of human functioning; (2) the diversity of data at a number of levels and from a variety of sources provides us with opportunities for validating and corroborating our impressions from any single source.

DEFINITIONS OF MENTAL HEALTH AND ILLNESS

Two additional problems remain to be considered. So far, in our discussion, we have refrained from addressing the issue of how the presence or absence of psychopathology is established in cross-cultural research. Indeed, in most of the research projects extant the cross-cultural assessor of psychopathology has entered the scene at the second stage of the proceedings. The decision of who is disturbed and who is not had already been made for the assessor, in part by professional personnel, in part by the patient's family and other community agents by directing him or her toward these services (Draguns, 1977b). As a result, the task of the mental health assessor in a cross-cultural project is to determine the kind of psychopathology the patient is suffering from rather than establish its presence or absence.

An exception to this general rule is established in cases of epidemiological studies, especially where the investigator comes from outside the culture to conduct a psychiatric census (for example, see Bash & Bash-Liechti, 1969). The baselines for the determination of psychological disturbance have been notoriously variable in research of this type, leading a number of reviewers of this kind of research to conclude that substantive and definitive conclusions could not be drawn from the aggregate of these findings (Dohrenwend & Dohrenwend, 1974; Marsella, 1979; Mariategui & Adis Castro, 1970). As a corrective to possible arbitrariness of such external determination of psychopathology, a few epidemiological inves-tigators explicitly sought and incorporated the judgment of local consultants and informants into their diagnoses of psychological disorder (see Bash & Bash-Liechti, 1969; Leighton et al., 1963). In the overwhelming majority of studies, the determination of a diagnos-able psychological disturbance is made by experts from within the culture. Implicitly, a consensus appears to be operating that, while neither the outsider's nor the insider's perspective affords a perfect view, insiders are preferable to outsiders in matters of psychiatric diagnosis. It is virtually universally, although tacitly, recognized that both knowledge of abnormal behavior patterns and familiarity with the culture in which they occur are prerequisites for the effective practice of psychiatric diagnosis. The advantage of an unprepossessed view that a person from outside the culture might bring is offset by the potential for misunderstanding the meaning and significance of acts in their cultural context. In the elegant phrase of Portuguese psychiatrist Barahona-Fernandes (1971), "Psychological disorder is personality in a situation." The external observer may lack enough information on, or familiarity with, the situation to fit all the pieces of the evidence properly at the service of diagnostic assignment.

The second issue pertains to the assessment of mental health, a topic explicitly mentioned in the title of this chapter. So far, nothing has been said about it and this is not accidental. Retracing the footsteps in the development of psychiatric assessment in culturally homogeneous milieus, substantive and methodological evaluation across cultures has been lopsidedly concentrated upon disturbance and dysfunction rather than upon their opposites. This activity represents the gist of the practical effort of mental health professionals as part of their mission.

Moreover, it will have been noticed that most of the prominent cross-cultural research projects of psychopathological populations have been concentrated selectively upon the most serious kinds of psychopathology—schizophrenia and affective disorders. It is no accident that there is as yet no World Health Organization international study on anxiety disorders or on the passive aggressive personality. Apart from the practical and clinical urgency of the effort of understanding the most serious patterns of human dysfunction on a world wide basis, the reason for this selective preoccupation with nonambulatory disorders is to be sought in the ease with which these disorders are spotted and identified in any cultural milieu.

The pronounced cultural relativism applied to the problem of psychological disorders (see Benedict, 1934) has given way to the realization that the most serious varieties of psychological disorders are recognized and indigenously labeled in most, if not all, cultures of the world (Murphy, 1976; see also Draguns, 1980). It is difficult for a culture to stand by in the face of the extremes of deviation in cognitive, affective, and social functioning. Thus comparative research in the range of functional psychoses can proceed on the basis of minimal definitions of disturbance and normality emanating from within cultures. These definitions are largely consensual across cultures. Such, however, is not the case as we proceed to a more demanding determination of mental health and mental illness and, in particular, to the so-called definitions of positive mental health, as exemplified by the listing of characteristics necessary for fully adequate functioning proposed by Jahoda (1958). The perusal of this well-known listing—featuring such characteristics as self-acceptance, ability for growth, development, and self-actualization, capacity for integration, sense of autonomy, perception of reality, and environmental mastery—makes it clear that it reflects, in part, widely shared values in our culture. Thus, in the case of other cultures characterized by a less rapid pace of social change than ours, less value might be placed on environmental mastery and autonomy and more on fitting into a supraordinate social unit—such as family, community, and state.

In cultures characterized by a passive premise in response to stress (Diaz Guerrero, 1967; Holtzman, Diaz Guerrero, & Swartz, 1975), greater values might be placed on adapting to, as opposed to mastering and confronting and subduing, what are perceived as the immutable features of the physical and social environment. Various definitions of positive mental health that have been proposed so far represent basically the culturally shared notions of a good life. As such, these statements are of necessity grounded in the values and the implicit or explicit philosophies of life of a given culture. If research based on these notions is ever attempted, it should proceed from a careful conceptual analysis of the philosophical sources of these definitions. Better yet, notions of positive mental health originating in several cultural traditions might be formulated, compared, and incorporated into comparative research across cultures. Before these concepts are applied to the participants of the study, the notions of positive mental health of mental professionals of different cultures might be articulated and compared. This, as yet, has not been attempted on a multicultural scale. The studies by Townsend (1975a, 1975b, 1978) comparing the United States and Germany in attitudes toward mental illness do not bear directly on values and conceptions of optimal functioning. This research, however, has contributed the interesting finding, worth extending and replicating, that attitudes toward and conceptions of mental illness run parallel in groups of patients, laypersons, and psychiatrists within a culture. The same state of affairs might conceivably be uncovered in relation to the more fundamental issue of what the optimal patterns of behavior are within a culture.

CONCLUSIONS

The points made in this chapter can now be restated and summarized as follows.

(1) The most typical and successful approach to comparison of psychologically disturbed individuals in several cultures has been by means of standardized verbal instruments of appraisal, exemplified by symptom rating scales, filled out by the patient, the psychiatrist, or a friend or associate of the patient.

(2) This development has made it possible to gather findings that have helped correct misconceptions about the culturally characteristic patterns of psychological disorder, such as in the case of the United States and Great Britain. It has also permitted the emergence of data pointing to a functional relationship between the course of the

disorder and antecedent cultural characteristics, as in the case of the World Health Organization (1979) follow-up study (Cooper & Sartorious, 1977).

(3) The fast pace of these developments has outstripped the application of other means of appraisal in cross-cultural research. As a result, an imbalance has resulted toward etic conceptualization of disorder, emphasizing worldwide similarities and deemphasizing differences. The etic basis has gone hand in hand with an inadvertent neglect of the phenomenology of disturbed experience, psychodynamics, and generally subjective reactions. Yet there are reasons to believe that all of these are potentially valuable sources of data on the culturally influenced experience of psychopathology.

(4) Similarly, comparative experimental research on psychological characteristics (beyond symptoms) and on physiological reactivity has, so far, not been undertaken. Filling these gaps in our accumulation of findings is desirable for two reasons: (a) They may shed light on some as yet unresolved issues, such as worldwide distribution of depression; and (b) they might help us integrate the findings of research in these areas, pursued independently in several countries and, as yet, rarely compared in terms of their findings.

(5) Self-report psychological inventories are in ascendancy in cross-cultural research on psychological disturbance. The thrust of these studies is, however, often divergent from cross-cultural comparison of psychopathology as the tools need to be adapted in content and wording and become less comparable to the originals from which they have been derived.

(6) By comparison, projective techniques in the cross-cultural assessment of abnormal behavior are in a state of neglect and decline. It is contended that their usefulness as ancillary and complementary sources of data on psychopathology across cultures has not been refuted; rather, it has never been put to a systematic and conclusive test.

(7) To counteract the dominance of the etic research strategy in this field, a four-step sequence, following Marsella (1978), is proposed. It begins with an emically based data collection and converts these data into potentially etic dimensions through the use of multivariate techniques of data analysis.

(8) For valid conceptual and practical reasons, the field of cross-cultural assessment has been almost entirely restricted to disorder, to the exclusion of mental health. In the field of disorder, most of the

assessment and research effort has been focused upon the most serious and conspicuous disorders on the determination of which there is a general consensus. Extension of this research to milder varieties of psychological disorder hinges on the development of interculturally acceptable definitions of mental health. It is pointed out that the definitions of positive mental health found in the Western literature may not be valid or acceptable across culture lines.

(9) More generally, diversification in measures, concepts, and research strategies is recommended to bring to the fore the interplay of culture and psychopathology in all of its facets.

REFERENCES

Al-Issa, I. (1977). Social and cultural aspects of hallucination. *Psychological Bulletin, 84,* 570-587.

Al-Issa, I. (1978). Sociocultural factors in hallucinations. *Internal Journal of Social Psychiatry, 24,* 167-176.

Barahona-Fernandes, H. J. (1971). Modelo de procesamiento del diagnostico psiquiatrico. *Revista de Neuro-Psiquiatria* (Lima), *34,* 75-90.

Bash,, K.W., & Bash-Liechti, J. (1969). Studies of the epidemiology of neuropsychiatric disorders among the rural population of the province of Khuzestan, Iran. *Social Psychiatry, 4,* 137-143.

Benedict, R. (1934). Culture and the abnormal. *Journal of Genetic Psychology, 1,* 60-64.

Block, J. (1965). *The challenge of response sets.* New York: Appleton-Century-Crofts.

Boesch, E. E. (1971). *Zwischen zwei Wirklichkeiten: Prolegomena einer okologischen Psychologie.* Berne: Huber.

Boyer, L. B., Klopfer, B., Brawer, F. B., & Kawai, H. (1964). Comparisons of shamans and pseudoshamans of the Miscalero Indian reservation. *Journal of Projective Techniques, 28,* 173-180.

Brislin, R. W. (1970). Back-translation for cross-cultural research. *Journal of Cross-Cultural Psychology, 1,* 185-216.

Brislin, R. W. (Ed.). (1976). *Translation: Applications and research.* New York: John Wiley.

Butcher, J. N., & Clarke, L.A. (1978). Recent trends in cross-cultural MMPI research and application. In J. N. Butcher (Ed.), *New developments in the use of the MMPI.* Minneapolis: University of Minnesota Press.

Butcher, J.N., & Pancheri, P. (1975). *A handbook of cross-cultural MMPI research.* Minneapolis: University of Minnesota Press.

Cattell, R.B., & Scheier, I. H. (1961). *The meaning and measurement of neuroticism.* New York: Academic.

Chun, K., Campbell, J., & Yoo, J. (1974). Extreme response style in cross-cultural research: A reminder. *Journal of Cross-Cultural Psychology, 5*, 465-480.

Cohen, R. (1967). Eine Untersuchung zur diagnostischen Verarbeitung widerspruchlicher Information. *Psychologische Forschung, 30*, 211-225.

Cooper, J. E., Kendell, R. E., Gurland, B. J., Sharpe, L., Copeland, J.R.M., & Simon, R. (1972). *Psychiatric diagnosis in New York and London.* Oxford University Press.

Cooper, J.E., & Sartorius, N. (1977). Cultural and temporal variations in schizophrenia. *British Journal of Psychiatry, 130*, 50-55.

DeVos, G. A. (1965). Transcultural diagnosis of mental health by means of psychological tess. In A.V.S. DeReuck & R. Porter (Eds.), *Transcultural psychiatry.* Boston: Little, Brown.

DeVos, G. A. (1976). The relationship of social and psychological structures in transcultural psychiatry. In W. P. Lebra (Ed.), *Culture-bound syndromes, ethnopsychiatry, and alternate therapies.* Honolulu: University Press of Hawaii.

Diaz Guerrero, R. (1967). Sociocultural premises, attitudes, and cross-cultural research. *International Journal of Psychology, 2*, 79-88.

Dinges, N. G., Trimble, J. E., Manson, S. M., & Pasquale, F. L. (1981). Counseling and psychotherapy with American Indians and Alaskan natives. In A. J. Marsella & P. B. Pedersen (Eds.), *Cross-cultural counseling and psychotherapy.* Elmsford, NY: Pergamon.

Diop, M. (1967). La depression chez le noir africain. *Psychopathologie Africaine, 3*, 183-194.

Dohrenwend, B. P., & Dohrenwend, B. S. (1974). Social and cultural influences upon psychopathology. *Annual Review of Psychology, 25*, 419-452.

Doi, T. (1973). *The anatomy of dependence* (J. Bester, Trans.). Tokyo: Kodansha.

Draguns, J. G. (1973). Comparisons of psychopathology across cultures: Issues, findings, directions. *Journal of Cross-Cultural Psychology, 4*, 9-47.

Draguns, J. G. (1977a). Advances in methodology of cross-cultural psychiatric assessment. *Transcultural Psychiatric Research Review, 14*, 125-143.

Draguns, J. G. (1977b). Problems of defining and comparing abnormal behavior across cultures. *Annals of the New York Academy of Sciences, 285*, 664-675.

Draguns, J. G. (1979a). Cultura y personalidad. In J. O. Whittaker (Ed.), *La psicological social en el mundo de hoy.* Mexico City: Trillas.

Draguns, J. G. (1979b). Culture and personality. In A. J. Marsella, R. Tharp, & T. J. Ciborowski (Eds.), *Perspectives on cross-cultural psychology.* New York: Academic.

Draguns, J. G. (1979c). Culture and personality: Old field, new directions. In L. H. Eckensberger, W. J. Lonner, & Y. Poortinga (Eds.), *Cross-cultural contributions to psychology: Selected papers from the IV International Conference of I.A.C.C.P.* Amsterdam: Swets & Zeitlinger.

Draguns, J. G. (1980). Psychological disorders of clinical severity. In H. C. Triandis & J. G. Draguns (Eds.), *Handbook of cross-cultural psychology: Vol. 6. Psychopathology.* Boston: Allyn & Bacon.

Draguns, J. G. (1982). Methodology in cross-cultural psychopathology. In I. Al-Issa (Ed.), *Culture and psychopathology.* Baltimore: University Park Press.

Durojaiye, M.O.A. (1975). Patterns of anxiety among Ugandan adolescents. In J. Berry & W. Lonner (Eds.), *Applied cross-cultural psychology.* Amsterdam: Swets & Zeitlinger.

Endler, N. S., & Magnusson, D. (1976). Multidimensional aspects of state and trait anxiety: A cross-cultural study of Canadian and Swedish college students. In C. D. Spielberger & R. Diaz Guerrero (Eds.), *Cross-cultural anxiety.* Washington, DC: Hemisphere.

Engelsmann, F., Vinar, P., Pichot, P., Hippius, H., Giberti, F., Rossi, L., & Overall, J. E. (1971). International comparison of diagnostic patterns. *Transcultural Psychiatric Research Review, 7,* 130-137.

Fabrega, H. J. (1974). *Disease and social behavior: An interdisciplinary perspective.* Cambridge: MIT Press.

Fabrega, H. J., & Silver, D. B. (1973). *Illness and shamanistic curing in Zinacantan: An ethnomedical analysis.* Stanford, CA: Stanford University Press.

Finifter, B. M. (1977). The robustness of cross-cultural findings. *Annals of the New York Academy of Sciences, 285,* 151-184.

Gauron, E. F., & Dickinson, J. K. (1966). Diagnostic decision making in psychiatry II. Diagnostic styles. *Archives of General Psychiatry, 14,* 233-237.

Gorham, D. R. (1970). Cross-cultural research based on the Holtzman Inkblot Technique. *Proceedings of the Seventh International Congress of the Rorschach and Other Projective Techniques,* pp. 158-164.

Hamilton, M. (1967). Development of a rating scale for primary depressive illness. *British Journal of Social and Clinical Psychology, 6,* 278-296.

Holtzman, W. H. (1980. Projective techniques. In D. C. Triandis & J. W. Berry (Eds.), *Handbook of cross-cultural psychology: Vol. 2. Methodology.* Boston: Allyn & Bacon.

Holtzman, W. H., Diaz Guerrero, R., & Swartz, J. D. (1975). *Personality development in two cultures.* Austin: University of Texas Press.

Jahoda, M. (1958). *Current concepts of positive mental health.* New York: Basic Books.

Joyce, C.R.B. (1980). Cultural variations in the response to pharmacotherapy and the "non-specific" factors which may affect this or "We know all the answers—it is the questions that we do not know." *Transcultural Psychiatric Research Review, 17,* 129-148.

Katz, M. M., Sanborn, K. O., Lowery, H. A., & Ching, J. (1978). Ethnic studies in Hawaii: On psychopathology and social deviance. In L. C. Wynne, R. L. Cromwell, & S. Mathysse (Eds.), *The nature of schizophrenia: New approaches to research and treatment.* New York: John Wiley.

Kendell, R.E. (1973). Psychiatric diagnoses: A study of how they are made. *British Journal of Psychiatry, 122,* 437-445.

Kimura, B. (1965). Vergleichende Untersuchungen uber depressive Erkrankungen in Japan und Deutschland. *Fortschritte der Psychiatrie und Neurologie, 33,* 202-215.

Kimura, B. (1967) Phanomenologie des Schulderlebnisses in einer vergleichenden psychiatrischen Sicht. *Aktuelle Fragen der Psychiatrie und Neurologie, 6,* 54-65.

Kimura, B. (1972). Mitmenschlichkeit in der Psychiatrie. *Zeitschrift fur Klinische Psychologie, 20,* 3-13.

Kleinman, A. (1977). Depression, somatization, and the "new cross-cultural psychiatry." *Social Science and Medicine, 11,* 3-9.

Langner, T. S. (1962). A twenty-two item screening score of psychiatric symptoms indicating impairment. *Journal of Health and Human Behavior, 3,* 269-276.

Lasry, J. C. (1975). Multi-cultural comparisons of a mental health scale. In J. W. Berry & W. J. Lonner (Eds.), *Applied cross-cultural psychology*. Amsterdam: Swets & Zeitlinger.

Lasry, J. C. (1977). Cross-cultural perspective on mental health and immigrant adaptation. *Social Psychiatry, 12,* 49-55.

Leighton, A. H., Lambo, T. A., Hughes, C. C., Leighton, D. C., Murphy, J. M., & Macklin, D. B. (1963). *Psychiatric disorders among the Yoruba*. Ithaca, NY: Cornell University Press.

Leighton, D. C., Hagnell, O., Kellert, S. R., Leighton, A. H., Harding, J. S., & Danley, R. A. (1971). Psychiatric disorder in a Swedish and a Canadian community: An exploratory study. *Social Science and Medicine, 5,* 189-209.

Lindzey, G. (1961). *Projective techniques and cross-cultural research*. New York: Appleton-Century-Crofts.

Lorr, M. (Ed.). (1966). *Explorations in typing psychotics*. New York: Bergman.

Lorr, M., & Klett, J. C. (1968). Major psychiatric disorders: A cross-cultural study. *Archives of General Psychiatry, 19,* 652-658.

Lorr, M., & Klett, C. J. (1969a). Cross-cultural comparison of psychotic syndromes. *Journal of Abnormal Psychology, 74,* 531-545.

Lorr, M., & Klett, J. C. (1969b). Psychotic behavior types: A cross-cultural comparison. *Archives of General Psychiatry, 20,* 592-598.

Mariategui, J., & Adis Castro, G. (Eds.). (1970). *Epidemiologia psiquiatrica en America latina*. Buenos Aires: Fondo para la salud mental.

Marsella, A. J. (1978). Thoughts on cross-cultural studies on the epidemiology of depression. *Culture, Medicine, and Psychiatry, 2,* 343-357.

Marsalla, A. J. (1979). Cross-cultural studies of mental disorders. In A. J. Marsella, R. G. Tharp, & T. J. Ciborowski (Eds.), *Perspectives on cross-cultural psychology*. New York: Academic.

Marsella, A. J. (1980). Depressive experience and disorder across cultures. In H. C. Triandis & J. G. Draguns (Eds.), *Handbooks of cross-cultural psychology: Vol. 2. Methodology*. Boston: Allyn & Bacon.

Marsella, A. J., & Sanborn, K. (1973). *The comprehensive depressive symptom checklist*. Honolulu: Institute of Behavioral Sciences.

Marsella, A. J., Tanaka-Matsumi, J., & Sanborn, K. (1974). *Baselines of depressive symptomatology among normal Japanese-Nationals, Japanese-Americans, and Caucasian-Americans*. Unpublished manuscript, University of Hawaii, Honolulu.

Minkowski, E. (1966). *Traite de psychopathologie*. Paris: Presses Universitaries de France.

Murphy, H.B.M. (1969). Handling the culture dimension in psyciatric research. *Social Psychiatry, 4,* 11-15.

Murphy, H.B.M. (1972a). History and the evolution of syndromes: The striking case of latah and amok. In M. Hammer, K. Salzinger, & S. Sutton (Eds.), *Psychopathology*. New York: John Wiley.

Murphy, H.B.M. (1972b). Psychopharmacologie et variations ethno-culturelles. *Confrontations Psychiatriques, 9,* 163-185.

Murphy, H.B.M., & Raman, A. C. (1971). The chronicity of schizophrenia in indigenous tropical proples: Results of a twelve-year follow-up in Mauritius. *British Journal of Psychiatry, 118,* 489-497.

Murphy, J. M. (1976). Psychiatric labeling in cross-cultural perspective. *Science, 191,* 1019-1028.

Norton, W. A. (1967). A review of psychiatric rating scales. *Canadian Psychiatric Association Journal, 12,* 563-574.

Olatowura, M. O. (1973). The problem of diagnosing depression in Nigeria. *Psychopathologie africaine, 9,* 389-403.

Opler, M. K., & Singer, J. L. (1959). Ethnic differences in behavior and psychopathology: Italian and Irish. *International Journal of Social Psychiatry, 2,* 11-23.

Overall, J. E., & Gorham, D. R. (1962). The Brief Psychiatric Rating Scale. *Psychological Reports, 10,* 799-812.

Phillips, L., & Draguns, J. G. (1971). Classification of the behavior disorders. *Annual Review of Psychology, 22,* 447-482.

Prince, R., & Mambour, W. (1967). A technique for improving linguistic equivalence in cross-cultural surveys. *International Journal of Social Psychiatry, 13,* 229-327.

Rabin, A. I., Doneson, S. L., & Jentons, R. L. (1979). Studies of psychological functions in schizophrenia. In L. Bellak (Ed.), *Disorders of the schizophrenic syndrome.* New York: Basic Books.

Raman, A. C., & Murphy, H.B.M. (1972). Failure of traditional prognostic indicators of Afro-Asian psychotics: Results of a long-term follow-up study, *Journal of Nervous and Mental Disease, 154,* 238-247.

Rorer, L. G. (1965). The great response style myth. *Psychological Bulletin, 63,* 129-148.

Scheff, T. J. (1966). *Being mentally ill: A sociological theory.* Chicago: Aldine.

Scheper-Hughes, N. (1979). *Saints, scholars, and schizophrenics: Mental illness in rural Ireland.* Berkeley: University of California Press.

Sechrest, L., Fay, T., & Zaidi, S. (1972). Problems of translation in cross-cultural research. *Journal of Cross-Cultural Psychology, 3,* 41-56.

Sharma, S. (1977). Cross-cultural comparisons of anxiety: Methodological problems. *Topics in culture Learning, 5,* 166-173.

Spain, D. H. (1972). On the use of projective techniques in psychological anthropology. In F.L.K. Hsu (Ed.), *Psychological anthropology* (rev. ed.). Cambridge, MA: Schenkman.

Spielberger, C.A., & Diaz Guerrero, R. (Eds.). (1976). *Cross-cultural anxiety.* Washington, DC: Hemisphere.

Spitzer, R. L., Endicott, J., Fleiss, J., & Cohen, J. (1970). The Psychiatric Status Schedule: A technique for evaluating psychopathology and impairment of role functioning. *Archives of General Psychiatry, 23,* 41-55.

Spitzer, R. L., & Fleiss, J. (1974). A reanalysis of the reliability of psychiatric diagnosis. *British Journal of Psychiatry, 125,* 341-347.

Stewart, E. C. (1981). Cultural sensitivities in counseling. In P. B. Pedersen, J. G. Draguns, W. J. Lonner, & J. E. Trimble (Eds.), *Counseling across cultures* (rev. ed.). Honolulu: University Press of Hawaii.

Tan, E. K., & Carr, J. E. (1977). Psychiatric sequelae of amok. *Culture, Medicine, and Psychiatry, 1,* 59-67.

Tanaka-Matsumi, J. (1979). Taijin-kyofusho: Diagnostic and cultural issues in Japanese psychiatry. *Culture, Medicine, and Psychiatry, 3,* 231-245.

Tanaka-Matsumi, J., & Marsella, A. J. (1976). Cross-cultural variations in the phenomenological experience of depression. *Journal of Cross-Cultural Psychology, 7,* 379-396.

Tanaka-Matsumi, J., & Marsella, A. J. (1977). *Ethnocultural variations in the subjective experience of depression: Semantic differential.* Unpublished manuscript, University of Hawaii, Honolulu.

Tapp, J. L. (1981). Personality development. In H. C. Triandis, A. Heron, & E. Kroeger (Eds.), *Handbook of cross-cultural psychology: Vol. 4. Developmental psychology.* Boston: Allyn & Bacon.

Tellenbach, H. (1972). Das Problem des Massstabls in der transkulturellen Psychiatrie. *Nervenarzt, 43,* 424-426.

Tellenbach, H. (1976). *Melancholie.* Heidelberg: Springer.

Torrey, E. F. (1972). *The mind game: Witchdoctors and psychiatrists.* New York: Emerson Hall.

Townsend, J. M. (1975a). Cultural conceptions, mental disorders, and social roles: A comparison of Germany and America. *American Sociological Review, 40,* 739-752.

Townsend, J. M. (1975b) Cultural conceptions and mental illness: A controlled comparison of Germany and America. *Journal of Nervous and Mental Disease, 160,* 409-421.

Townsend, J. M. (1978). *Cultural conceptions of mental illness.* Chicago: University of Chicago Press.

Triandis, H. C. (1972). *The analysis of subjective culture.* New York: John Wiley.

Triandis, H. C. (1977). Cross-cultural social and personality psychology. *Personality and Social Psychology Bulletin, 3,* 143-158.

Vassiliou, G., & Vassiliou, V. (1974). Subjective culture and psychotherapy. *American Journal of Psychotherapy, 28,* 566-573.

Villeneuve, A. (1970). Classification des medicaments psychotropes, nosologie et echelles d'appreciation. *Canadian Psychiatric Association Journal, 15,* 205-213.

Wagatsuma, H. (1977). Problems of language in cross-cultural research. *Annals of the New York Academy of Sciences, 285,* 141-150.

Waxler, N. E. (1979). Is outcome of schizophrenia better in nonindustrial societies? The case of Sri Lanka. *Journal of Nervous and Mental Disease, 167,* 144-158.

Wing, J. K., Cooper, J. E., & Sartorius, N. (1974). *Measurement and classification of psychiatric symptoms.* Cambridge: Cambridge University Press.

Wittenborn, J. R. (1972). Reliability, validity, and objectivity of symptom-rating scales. *Journal of Nervous and Mental Disease, 154,* 79-82.

Wohl, O. J. (1981). Intercultural psychotherapy: Issues, questions, and reflections. In P. B. Pedersen, J. G. Draguns, W. J. Lonner, & J. E. Drimble (Eds.), *Counseling across cultures* (rev. ed.). Honolulu: University Press of Hawaii.

World Health Organization. (1973). *Report of the International Pilot Study of Schizophrenia.* Geneva: Author.

World Health Organization. (1979). *Schizophrenia: An international follow-up study.* New York: John Wiley.

Yap, P. M. (1974). *Comparative psychiatry: A theoretical framework.* Toronto: University of Toronto Press.

Zeldine, G., Ahvi, R., Leuckx, R., Boussat, M., Saibou, A., Hanck, C., Collignon, R., Tourame, G., & Collomb, H. (1975). A propos de l'utilisation d'une echelle d'evaluation en psychiatrie transculturelle. *L'Encephale, 1,* 133-145.

Zubin, J. (1967). Classification of the behavior disorders. *Annual Review of Psychology, 18*, 373-406.

Zung, W. (1969). A cross-cultural survey of symptoms of depression. *American Journal of Psychiatry, 126*, 116-121.

Zung, W. (1972). A cross-cultural survey of depressive symptomatology in normal adults. *Journal of Cross-Cultural Psychology, 3*, 177-183.

3

SHAMANS AND ENDORPHINS
Exogenous and Endogenous Factors in Psychotherapy

RAYMOND PRINCE

In 1974, Harry Triandis asked me to contribute a chapter on psychotherapy to his *Handbook of Cross-Cultural Psychology*. I faced this task with a heavy heart. It was not that the subject is inherently dull. On the contrary, the variety of richness of the field is highly exciting—a veritable chest of jewels for any psychological or anthropological fortune hunter. My problem was that the subject had been worked over repeatedly by such perceptive authors as Frank (1961), Kiev (1964), and Torry (1972), to mention only the best known, and although there was a steadily increasing volume of descriptions of culture-bound forms of therapy, the same universal therapeutic factors were being cited repeatedly: the shared world view, labeling of the disease and attribution of cause, the expectations of the patient, and the central role of suggestion. Many of these writings had also a marked polemical flavor attacking psychoanalysis. Ritualistically, the authors concluded their descriptions with the same recitation of factors and the same polemics. The problem was not that the individual jewels lacked luster, but that the mountings had become hackneyed.

As I was reviewing definitions of psychotherapy, however, I came upon Frank's (1961, p.1) formulation:

> Attempts to enhance a person's feeling of well being are usually labelled treatment, and every society trains some of its members to apply this form of influence. Treatment always involves a *personal relationship between healer and sufferer.* Certain types of therapy rely primarily on the *healer's ability to mobilize healing forces in the sufferer* by psychological means. These forms of treatment may be generically termed psychotherapy. (italics added)

Two points struck me in this definition. The first was that treatment always involved the healer-patient dyad. This point was striking because I had just returned from a visit to India, where I had observed a healing ceremony without a healer! In Lucknow, a large group of patients knelt at sundown before the ancient shrine of a deceased Islamic saint. Patients became violently possessed during a half-hour period. Most were required (on the basis of instructions issued by the possessing spirit to relatives of the patient who were in attendance) to present themselves at the shrine on thirty consecutive evenings to be healed. According to the local populace, the ceremony had been practiced from time immemorial and a good proportion of the supplicants recovered from their illnesses (Prince, 1980). The other important point in Frank's (1961) definition was the idea that there were endogenous healing factors that the healer was able to mobilize. Frank was of course referring to the mobilization of expectation and hope. A combination of both points suggested that more attention should be devoted to endogenous processes in the explanation of healing. The recoveries before the Islamic shrine must result largely from the mobilization of hope and other endogenous mechanisms. Perhaps the influence of the healer is not always as important as Frank and others have believed.

Following this line of reasoning, I developed the idea that there were two fundamental healing components in psychotherapeutic systems: (1) the much-discussed exogenous factors, such as shared world views, suggestion, and so forth, which derive largely from the healer and the culture; and (2) the endogenous factors that derive largely from the patients themselves. In considering this latter group of factors, the question to be asked was what individuals themsleves do under stressful circumstances and what spontaneous phenomena occur to them as a result of their own biological organization and defenses. Some go to sleep or withdraw and rest; some try to puzzle out a solution to the stressful problems; others may socialize, go on a drinking spree, or buy a new hat or horse; less commonly, they may deprive or punish themselves or make a suicidal gesture. On the other hand, involuntary coping mechanisms may come into play; they may dream about the problem, or be subject to a religious experience or psychotic episode. In this context, I argued that healers around the world have learned to manipulate and elaborate upon a number of these endogenous mechanisms, including sleep, dreams, dissociated states, religious experiences, and psychoses in a variety of ways to bring about resolution of life problems and alleviation of suffering (Prince, 1976).

As I was working with these ideas, the first descriptions of exciting new developments in neurochemistry began to appear. These had to do with the discovery of the endorphins, or endogenously generated morphinelike substances. In a remarkable display of scientific creativity, literally hundreds of papers on various aspects of the endorphins have appeared in the past few years (for reviews, see Cleghorn, 1979; Guillemin, 1978; Kosterlitz & Hughes, 1977; Snyder, 1978). The spark that ignited these pyrotechnics was the discovery that neurons in diverse areas of the nervous system were equipped with receptor sites that accepted only levorotary opiate molecules. But why should such receptor sites have evolved when very few organisms have ever been exposed to substances that were thought to be produced exclusively by the opium poppy? Clearly, it was sensible to suppose that there must also be endogenously generated molecules that were similar in configuration and effects to morphine. The quest for the endogenous morphinelike substance was on. Hughes et al. (1975) discovered two five-chain amino-acid compounds (met-enkephalin and leu-enkephalin) that showed the appropriate characteristics. Almost simultaneously, a longer chain molecule (beta-endorphin) with morphinelike properties was discovered.

Although the study of the significance of these substances has only just begun, it is highly probable that they are of fundamental biopsychological importance. For our present purposes, only some of the findings that might be related to endogenous healing mechanisms will be mentioned. As regards the functions of the endorphins, most work has been done on their pain-relieving effects. The following phenomena have been found to be mediated in whole or in part by the endorphins: the analgesic effects of electrical self-stimulation of brain electrode implants used for the treatment of chronic intractable pain (Akil, Richardson, & Barchas, 1979); surgical anaesthesia produced by acupuncture (Mayer, Price, & Raffi, 1977) and the pain relief for a wide variety of injuries and illnesses afforded by transcutaneous stimulation (Chapman & Benedetti, 1977); and the naturally occurring analgesia of those rather rare individuals who suffer congenital absence of pain perception (Dehen, Willer, Boureau, & Cambier, 1977). Exorphins (as the opiates from the opium poppy are now called) also produce amnesia for pain and for unpleasant events. It has been found that endorphins produce similar amnesia in rats (Messing et al., 1979). Little work has been done on the euphoria-producing aspects of opiates, but Belluzzi and Stein (1977) have found that rats will repeatedly bar-press in Skinner boxes to receive microinjections of met- and leu-enkephalin delivered directly into their own cerebral ventricles. This bar-pressing effect is blocked by naloxone (a morphine antagonist), suggesting that the reward system, presumably rat euphoria, is activated by endorphins. The role of endorphins in alterations of consciousness has not yet been investigated.

If these are some of the functions of the endorphins, we must next ask how they are generated. There is a considerable body of research suggesting that endorphins are released under circumstances of physical stress and concomitant with other well-known stress hormones, such as ACTH. For example, they have been found to be elevated significantly in blood as a result of intense muscular activity such as long-distance running or other strenuous exercise (Appenzeller, Standefer, Appenzeller, & Atkinson, 1980; Carr, Bullen & Skrinar, 1981). There is also some evidence that psychological stress releases endorphins. This is a more difficult research area because it is difficult to identify situations that are psychologically stressful for an animal but that are not at the same time physically stressful. As far as human research is concerned, the use of situations representing genuine psychological threat often presents serious ethical problems. Pert (1981) has described an experiment with rats that seems to implicate psychological stress. Rats respond to repeated painful stimuli by showing an increase in endorphin-related analgesia. When the same rats are subsequently placed in the same shock chambers (but do not in fact receive shocks), they once again show elevations in endorphins and pain thresholds. These latter elevations were felt to be in response to conditioned fear, which is a kind of psychological stress. Clearly, further research linking endorphins and psychological stress should have a high priority.

To summarize, there is now considerable experimental and circumstantial evidence that endogenously generated neurohormones produce analgesia, euphoria, amnesia, and altered states of consciousness, all of which are also generated by religious and other rituals that constitute an important element in many endogenous psychotherapeutic systems.

These discoveries present something of a problem for the evolutionary minded. The question is, why should the organism provide two mechanisms that seem to nullify one another? On the one hand, there are well-developed pain and fear systems that have high survival value. On the other hand, endorphin research suggests that there is also an antagonistic system that alleviates pain and fear. A possible resolution of this contradiction would seem to be that pain and fear occur in situations of ordinary stress. But in some circumstances they can become maladaptive. When pain or fear is excessive or prolonged, it can prevent fight or flight. It seems reasonable to suppose that the endorphins, and possibly other anodyne and tranquilizing hormones, are released in circumstances of hyperarousal that may become maladaptive.

In this chapter, I will display endogenous healing institutions in a new light by linking them in a speculative way with this body of neuroendocrine research. Two hypothetical relationships will be presented that will attempt to link neurohormones with hyperarousal, and with what I have called the "omnipotence maneuver," a remarkable state of mind which is very common in endogenous healing phenomena.[1]

NEUROHORMONES AND HYPERAROUSAL

To introduce the concept of hyper- and hypoarousal, I will first mention the work on film-induced stress by Levi (1972) and his group at the World Health Organization stress laboratories in Stockholm. Levi showed male and female students a selection of films that were judged to be bland, humorous, terrifying, anger provoking, and sexually explicit. As measures of emotional arousal, he used self-reports and measures of sympathoadrenomedullary activity including urinary volume and urinary excretion of adrenaline, noradrenaline, and creatinine. It was found that the bland films (natural scenery, which elicited self-reports of boredom) produced significant reductions in the biological arousal measures, whereas the anger, fear, humor, and sexually arousing films produced significant increases in the same measures. Globus and Shulman (1963) had earlier called attention to the fact that films were valuable in experimental induction of emotional reactions because the darkness, immobility, relative lack of distractions, and isolation from objective reality-oriented interpersonal events all facilitate the provocation of affective arousal.

Let us now turn to that much more archaic cinematographic display—the dream. I will first briefly review some of the well-known findings about dreams, most of which have emerged in the past twenty years since the germinal discovery of REM (rapid eye movement) sleep by Aserinsky and Kleitman (1953). Most typical dreams occur during REM sleep and, although everyone has four to five dream periods a night, the vast majority of dreams are forgotten. During REM sleep the motor system is disconnected; the sleeper is totally paralyzed and has absent tendon reflexes. During REM sleep (or, more specifically, during so-called phasic activities that predominate during REM sleep), a variety of physiological activities occur, including the twitching of the eye muscles (REMs) and of the middle-ear musculature, rapid pupilary size alterations, penile erections, cardiovascular irregularities, and widely distributed muscle twitches (for a review of these findings, see Dement & Mitler, 1975). During dreams, reality testing virtually disappears, so that the dreamer does not question the reality of the many impossible happenings that occur on the dream screen.

I would like to suggest, then, that we have an indwelling movie theater that potentially can display for us every night especially selected "films." These "films" can artificially elicit the whole range of hyper- or hypoarousal and the entire spectrum of human emotions from boredom to horror and any imaginable gratification of the bed or board. And if the ordinary movie theater is especially valuable for producing mock emotions because of the darkness, immobility, and isolation from obejctive reality, these factors are much more marked in the indwelling theater. The dreaming self is totally paralyzed and totally taken in by the images because of its lack of reality testing. And, of course, the "program director" for the indwelling theater is uniquely equipped to choose the "films" that will most horrify, sexually titillate, or bore the dreamer, for, if we accept the psychoanalytic view, this "director" has access to the dreamer's own unconscious needs and fears.

I think the potential relationship between these ideas and the endorphins (or other as yet undiscovered stress neuroendocrines) is clear enough. As we have previously noted, endorphins seem to be released in conditions of hyperstress in which pain and terror become maladaptive. We also have experimental evidence that films give rise to alterations in the neuroendocrine system. It seems possible, then, that the indwelling theater, by producing mock terror or anger or sexual activities, could provide the circumstances for hyperarousal and for stress-endocrine release. One might expect that hyperarousal dreams would be most called for when the individual is suffering severe life stress and the neuroendocrine release generated by a dreamer's horror, for example, of castration in his nocturnal dream, will suffice to provide the euphoria necessary to help him handle his waking quarrel with his wife.

Let us at last turn our attention to the main theme of this presentation: cross-cultural psychotherapeutic systems. Although many systems utilize dreams in a peripheral way (Prince, 1980), their manipulation as a central feature of such systems is relatively rare. Well-known examples include psychoanalysis, the Asclepian temple incubation in ancient Greece, the Senoi system described by Stewart (1969), and the Iroquois system (Wallace, 1967). The last will serve as an example of how dream manipulations illustrate the hyperarousal hypothesis.

The basic Iroquois concept holds that the soul harbors inborn wishes, which, if they are not fulfilled, will result in sickness or death. Such misfortune may affect only the dreamer, but may also be shared by the group to which the dreamer belongs. Whatever occurs in dreams must be reenacted during waking. Wallace (1967) provides many examples of hyperarousal-type artificial situations in Iroquois dreams that were subsequently enacted in reality. For example, a common dream was that the individual was being tortured and burned by his enemies. Upon awakening, the dreamer demanded that he be tied up and burned as a captive. This action would preclude a similar event in reality at the hands of his enemies. Wallace (1967) cites an example of burns suffered in this way that did not heal for months. Another dreamer reported a similar dream to his council of elders and, as a result,

> twelve or thirteen fires were lighted in the cabin where captives were burned, and torturers seized fire brands. The dreamer was burned; "he shrieked like a madman. When he avoided one fire, he at once fell into another." Naked, he stumbled around the fires three times, singed by one torch after another, while his friends repeated compassionately, "courage, my Brother, it is thus that we have pity on thee." Finally he darted out of the ring, seized a dog held for him there, and paraded through the cabins with this dog on his shoulders, publicly offering it as a consecrated victim of the demon of war, "begging him to accept this semblance instead of the reality of his Dream." The dog was finally killed with a club, roasted in the flames, and eaten at a public feast. (Wallace, 1967, p. 170)

We might also cite the example of a Cayuga man who dreamed that he gave a feast of human flesh. The tribal council believed that the dream had important implications for the whole group and to protect against disaster the dream must certainly be carried out. One of the counselor's brothers was offered for sacrifice to be cut up and placed in a kettle. The dreamer objected, pointing out that the victim must be a woman. A young woman was therefore adorned and delivered to the dreamer-executioner. Just as the fatal blow was to be delivered, the dreamer cried out, "I am satisfied, my dream requires nothing further" (Wallace, 1967, p. 180).

It is clear that most of the dreams and their waking realizations, cited by Wallace (1967), display hyperarousal situations involving self-damage, damage to others, sexual orgies, and so forth. Presumably, the Iroquois sometimes experienced more tranquil dreams. In any case, in the Iroquois system we see that the artificially induced hyperarousal of dreams is reenacted in real hyperarousal situations that involve not only the dreamer but also his fellow tribesmen. If we assume that such dreams would generate powerful endocrine reactions when displayed on the dream screen, they must also generate them when translated into reality, both for the dreamer and for his fellows. Wallace (1967) gives us no examples of deaths resulting from such reenactments so that, presumably, for the most part this therapeutic system, although often harsh, was adaptive given the Iroquois world view.

A much more widely distributed type of therapeutic system is that involving ritual dissociation states (also referred to as "possession" or "trance" states). These systems are particularly prominent in African cultures and in parts of the Americas populated by descendants of African slaves. But they are also to be found in India, Southeast Asia, the Middle East, and elsewhere (Bourguignon, 1968). These systems also lend themselves to discussion in terms of the hyperarousal hypothesis. Although they could very profitably be studied using the same technology as used to study sleep, dreams, sleepwalking, night terrors, narcolepsy, and so forth (Broughton, 1968), this has never been attempted. Some of the features of ritual dissociation states do indeed suggest a biological basis: (1) Induction is frequently achieved through dancing to music that features a pronounced and rapid beat; (2) induction frequently occurs following a period of starvation and/or a period of overbreathing; (3) the onset of dissociation is marked by a period of motor inhibition or collapse; (4) in the neophyte, collapse may be followed by a period of frenetic motor activity; once experience is acquired, a controlled diety-specific behavior pattern emerges; (5) during dissociation there is frequently a fine tremor of head and limbs; sometimes grosser, convulsive jerks occur; a diminution of sensory acuity may be evident; and (6) return to normal consciousness is followed by a sleep of exhaustion, from which the subject awakens in a state of mild euphoria and a more or less complete amnesia for the period of dissociation (Prince, 1968).

As an example of a therapeutic system of the dissociative type, I will briefly describe the medicine dance of the !Kung Bushman (Lee, 1968). This system is particularly relevant to the argument of this chapter because the !Kung emic explanation of their trances reads very much like a description of an endogenous therapeutic neuroendocrine system. They do not regard the dissociated state as resulting from mounting or possession by an alien spirit. Rather, they hold that all individuals have an indwelling medicine that is usually cool and inactive, but that is gradually brought to a "boil" in the medicine dance.

> Bushman medicine is put into the body through the backbone. It boils in my belly and boils up to my head, like beer. When the women start singing and I start dancing, at first I feel quite all right. Then in the middle, the medicine begins to rise from my stomach. After that, I see all the people like small birds. The whole place will be spinning around, and that is why we run around. The trees will be circling also. You feel your blood come very hot, just like blood boiling on a fire, and then you start healing. When I am like this [i.e., telling the story], I am just a person. The things comes up after a dance, then when I lay hands on a sick person, the medicine in me will go into him and cure him. (Lee, 1968, p. 43)

The medicine dance is an all-night affair. The trance dancers are all males; they dance in a wide circle of rhythmically clapping and chanting women who in turn are seated in a circle about a central fire. The dancers characteristically enter trance twice during the night, at about midnight and then again just before dawn.

As noted in the general description of dissociated states above, neophyte trancers behave in a wild and erratic way and often engage in fire walking or fire handling, running into the bush at top speed, attacking dogs, retching violently, acting out sexual intercourse, and attempting to expose their genitals. Older men restrain this dangerous or asocial behavior. As one informant reported:

> When I was first learning I stepped into the fire; now I am old and don't do it. The young ones in trance see the fires as if it is above their heads; they step in it because they think they are passing under it. When I stepped in fire I didn't burn my feet, because the medicine in my body is as hot as the fire; so when I stepped in I didn't get burned. . . . If I were to step in fire right now, when my medicine is cold, I would burn myself. (Lee, 1968, p. 43)

The !Kung also believe that human sweat generated during the medicine dance trances has a powerful therapeutic effect. Trancers rub the sweat from their bodies upon those who are ill and upon others to protect them from illness.

In these frenetic trance dances, we can perhaps see the same artificial hyperarousal phenomena as in some types of dreams. In trance, as in dreams, reality testing is grossly impaired. But trance hyperarousal behavior is probably a more powerful neuroendocrine stimulator than dreams since in trance the motor system is fully activated and the arousal more intense. It is possible that in frenetic trance behavior we can see both the stimulation of the neuroendocrine axis (the bringing of the medicine to a boil) and the analgesic and amnesic effects of these substances. Of course, it is clear that, as with dreams, not all trance behavior is artificially induced hyperarousal behavior. It is plausible that just as hyperarousal dreams are more common under circumstances of high life stress, so frenetic trance behavior is more marked and frequent with highly disturbed individuals and in highly stressful cultures. Some evidence for this is to be found when we compare the descriptions of voodoo possession phenomena (Metraux, 1959) in Haiti (a highly stressful regime) with the possession phenomena of Brazil (Leacock & Leacock, 1975). The distinct impression is gained that there is much less hyperaroused trance behavior in Brazil than in Haiti. The following description by Wittkower (1970, pp. 153-154) of a voodoo performance in Haiti is characteristic:

> Suddenly the *houngan* was seized by a state of possession. His face became expressionless, his eyes looked vacant, his mouth was half open, giving him a dull appearance and his head jerked forward and backward. At one time he put his big toe in his mouth, at another he fell

backward and had to be supported, at still another he struggled violently and had to be restrained. Eventually, in a state of exhaustion, he had to be carried into the *hounfort*. . . . At this point one of the women who had attracted our attention by her wild dancing movements reached a state of possession. Her movements became more and more seductive, her facial expression was one of blissful experience, and eventually in what amounted to an orgastic state she fell to the ground. As *Ghede,* the *loa* of Rabelaisian eroticism, was called on, the dancers hugged and clutched each other and pelvic movements of a crude, sexual nature dominated the scene. . . . Increasingly the crowd assumed a state of high sexual excitement which was driven to a still higher pitch by consumption of rum. By then a young man had passed into a state of possession displaying convulsive movements. A woman placed her head between the knees of a man, moving her body up and down rhythmically. Eventually the highest pitch was reached with the Marinette ceremony. Marinette is the *loa* of fire. A fire was lit in the yard adjoining the peristyle. It was fed by rum being poured on it, and the crowd in a state of frenzy danced around it. Men with long tubes which they blew cacophonously and beat with sticks joined the crowd, prancing backward and forward. The frenzied crowd exposed their limbs to the fire, some walked through it, and one man, rolling convulsively on the ground towards the fire, had to be prevented from being burned.

THE OMNIPOTENCE MANEUVER

Under some circumstances of life stress and artificially induced hyperarousal, the threatened individual may suddenly experience a profound sense of tranquillity. This flip-over from hyperarousal to euphoria is commonly linked with the idea of supernatural intervention (depending upon the world view of the subject) because the tranquillity arises without an externally visible reason—it arises from within as a kind of *deus ex machina.* This organic response to stress I will here designate as the "omnipotence manuever." In one form or another it is an all but universal feature of the endogenous healing mechanisms we are here considering.

A familiar example is to be found in some of the functional psychoses. In the context of highly stressful life circumstances, the response may be ego disintegration. The phenomenology of these states is well known and includes feelings of panic and world destruction and a loss of ego boundaries. Reality testing is grossly impaired.

In the midst of this *gotterdammerung,* there emerges a feeling of revelation and mastery associated with the delusion of ego omnipotence. The belief crystalizes that the psychotic is the savior of the world, the possessor of infinite truths, and so forth. With this certainty of omnipotence the hyperarousal state may revert to relative tranquillity and hypoarousal. Freud (1953) was perhaps the first to draw attention to this phenomenon when he pointed out that delusions should not be regarded as symptoms of illness but as attempts at self-healing.

In a lower key, we may also consider types of spontaneous religious experience, such as the mystical states described by James (1902), as examples of the omnipotence maneuver. Once again, these states often occur in circumstances of heightened life stress. The subject is visited by a brief ecstatic state with loss of ego boundaries, a certainty that the experience contains valid truths, and often the belief that the state has its origins in the divine.

We will use Koestler's (1954) description as an example. Koestler was sentenced to execution and imprisoned during the Spanish Civil War. He whiled away his time by working out mathematical puzzles on his prison wall. One day, on reaching the solution of a difficult problem, he was swept by a mystical experience?

> The significance of this swept over me like a wave. The wave had originated in an articulate verbal insight; but this evaporated at once, leaving it its wake only a wordless essence, a fragrance of eternity, a quiver of the arrow in the blue. I must have stood there for some minutes, entranced, with a wordless awareness that "this is perfect—perfect"; until I noticed some slight mental discomfort nagging at the back of my mind—some trivial circumstance that marred the perfection of the moment. Then I remembered the nature of that irrelevant annoyance: I was, of course, in prison and might be shot. But this was immediately answered by a feeling whose verbal translation would be: "So what? is that all? have you got nothing more serious to worry about?"—an answer so spontaneous, fresh and amused as if the intruding annoyance had been the loss of a collar-stud. Then I was floating on my back in a river of peace, under bridges of silence. It came from nowhere and flowed nowhere. Then there was no river and no I. The I had ceased to exist. (Koestler, 1954, p. 350)

Koestler subsequently received these experiences two or three times a week during the period of his imprisonment. It is interesting that he likens them to massive doses of vitamins injected into his veins. They left him with a serene and fear-dispelling aftereffect that lasted for hours or days. The long-term effect was that he developed a conviction of the existence of a supernatural order with attendant relief from his former fears and uncertainties.

Such experiences are evidently much more common than one might expect. Recent surveys in the United States and Britain suggest that some 20 percent to 40 percent of populations at large experience them, and some 5 percent experience them often (for a review, see Prince, 1979).

It is clear that this omnipotence maneuver is widely used in psychotherapeutic systems as a means to change beliefs and master fear. Evangelical preaching is one example that involves a charismatic religious leader who first evokes powerful feelings of sinfulness and individual worthlessness; at the height of this hyperarousal, the preacher holds out the possibility of salvation. Many subjects experience a flip-over to peace and tranquillity associated with a belief in divine forgiveness. A variety of "brainwashing" techniques and cult initiations employ similar methods. Freed (1980, p. 3) reports the following experience of a young man during his unplanned induction into the Unification Church (the Moonies cult). After several days of intense group pressure aimed at inducing powerful feelings of self-doubt and worthlessness,

> my head felt like it was splitting open from pressure, as though something inside me were swollen and about to burst. My adrenaline began pumping like I was being chased for my life and I was overflowing with anger, tension, confusion, and fear.

When he finally decided to stay with the cult, he felt as though "a huge weight had come off his shoulders and his body was gripped with a strange, disattached feeling. Electricity seemed to be pulsing through his veins in a buzzing sensation" (Freed, 1980, p. 10). That night he awoke and saw a brilliant white light. He shielded his eyes and the light enveloped him, "warming and soothing me, drawing the tension from my body." Then he fell into a perfect, tranquil sleep. When he awoke, he believed he had been sent a special signal telling him he was right to stay with the cult. He felt better than he had in days. His questions and doubts seemed to have faded, his fears and anxiety were gone.

I have already referred to the widespread use of dissociated states in therapeutic systems and have noted the fact that, characteristically, wild and excited behavior occurs during the early period of trancing. Subsequently, in many cults, this behavior calms down as a controlled deity-specific behavior emerges. The omnipotence maneuver manifests itself in the emic belief that this behavior represents the mounting or possession of the subject by appropriate deities. It is not clear, of course, what type of imagery is experienced by these subjects, either during their wild hyperaroused behavior or during their subsequent deity-specific behavior, since there is almost always amnesia for the dissociated episode. In many systems, controlled omnipotence behavior is displayed to the community in the form of dramatic performances with important religious functions. The following is a description of the public performance of the possessed members of the *Shopono* cult by the Yoruba of Nigeria (Prince, 1964, pp. 108-109):

> The main proceedings took place in the center of the village where a bamboo-and-palm roof had been made over an open space among the huts. Many large calabash bowls were laid out for sacrifice. These contained pounded yam balls, solidified pap, pieces of rope smeared with blook, the odd goat's head and some other unidentifiable objects. A pile of black sticks painted with red and white spots completed the array. The cult women, dressed alike in purple print cloth, were bustling about, as were a few male elders of the cult. The drumming had already begun, and there was an air of anticipation which heightneed as the drumming became more insistent. One of the cult members went among the people touching their heads with some pap to take away bad luck. The pap was put in one of the sacrificial bowls. There were many children standing about, round-eyed.

> Then the possession commenced. A knot of younger women collected about one tall old woman with a pock-marked face, all singing and moving to the drum beat. One girl stood before the old woman with her arms about her neck. They placed one of the sacrificial bowls upon the girl's head, and the women began to sing louder, calling upon the spirit of the particular *Sopono* that habitually possessed this girl. The girl's face became vacant, and her eyes focused upon a distant place. Suddenly she fell forward in a kind of swoon; the "mother" supported her; someone else seized the calabash so that it wouldn't fall; others threw water on her feet. In a few seconds she revived a little; they guided her fingers up over the rim of the calabash, and she was drawn to one side, where she stood, somewhat dazed, the "wife" of the god.

Ten or twelve other girls were possessed in the same way. Then in single file, bearing the sacrifices upon their heads, they commenced a slow dance about a tree in the center of the clearing. Finally they moved out in a procession about the whole village. Each householder splashed a little water and palm oil on the ground, and the possessed girls each dipped her foot in the pool and moved on. When all the bad luck and illness of the village had been collected in this way, the procession moved off, single file, to a place in the thick forest where sacrifices are deposited for *Sopono* beneath an ancient tree. The entire proceedings took about three hours.

I would suggest that just as group hyperarousal characterizes some of the reenacted dreams of the Iroquois system discussed previously, so group tranquillization may be an important effect of the public dramatic displays of divine intervention in the Yoruba example just cited. The community is reassured by the presence in their midst of the gods as guests.

Finally, I would like to draw attention to some of the psychotherapeutic systems that use micropsychoses produced by psychedelic plants as an example of the omnipotence maneuver. The use of psychedelics in this way is a central feature of many Amerindian systems, but is also found among groups in Siberia, Australia, and New Guinea (Dobkin de Rios, 1976). The Yanomamo of the upper Orinoco are heavy users of the dimethyltryptamine-containing snuff called *epena*. The powder the inner bark of the epena tree and blow it up one another's nostrils to produce the intoxication. Seitz (1967, pp. 329-330) describes the response as follows:

After inhaling the two doses of Epena, the usual quantity of snuff powder at the beginning of the ceremony, the Indian continued for about two or three minutes in his cowered position. Then he stood up and walked swaying like a drunkard. On his way his walk became faster and steadier. His stare became fixed and he experienced a violent perspiration. In a few minutes his face and body were completely wet.

Then his steps changed into a stamping that generally was adapted to a certain rhythm: three or four steps forward, one step on the same place. This "dance" the man accompanied with a recitative, monotonous singing, which was relieved about every five to eight minutes by a terrible yell. During this yelling the man generally stopped his "dance" and turned himself with high lifted or spread arms to the mountain-range that elevates itself, steep in the sky, a few miles to the north of the villages. . . .

The Indian feels that he is a giant; everything around him takes enormous and magnificent forms. In the midst of a super-dimensional world, he feels like a superman! Consequently, his movements correspond to this state of excitation. These are braggart's gestures. These symptoms are accompanied by profuse salivation, a bad headache, a fixed stare and heavy perspiration. The symptoms reveal a state of strong intoxication.

Is it possible to link this so-called omnipotence maneuver with neuroendocrine effects? The hypothesis that the omnipotence maneuver emerges when a critical level of endogenous euphoriant substances are generated suggests itself. As we have seen, the series of events leading up to the omnipotence manuever is usually as follows: (1) a situation of life stress; (2) this situation is exaggerated by mock displays in dreams of psychosis, or sometimes by the manipulations of healers; (3) in any case, a state of excessive hyperarousal occurs, which generates appropriate endorphins or other neuroendocrines in such quantities that an unprecedented feeling of cosmic peace and tranquillity is experienced, which is interpreted by the subject as resulting from supernatural agencies of some sort. It could also be suggested that perhaps because of the structural analogy between psychedelic drugs and endogenously produced neuroendocrines, the omnipotence effect may be produced simply by the ingestion of psychedelics without benefit of life stress, mock hyperarousal, or healers (as, for example, in the case of the epena users mentioned previously).

SUMMARY AND CONCLUSIONS

I have discussed a variety of endogenous healing mechanisms such as dreams, dissociated states, religious experiences, and micropsychoses that may emerge spontaneously in circumstances of life stress, or may be manipulated and developed by healers. I have attempted to show that it is possible to some extent to link these mechanisms with the possible functioning of the recently discovered endogenous morphinelike substances.

These neuroendocrines seem to be generated in situations of excessively intense or prolonged arousal, where they may nullify the usually adaptive reactions of pain and fear. That is, the endorphins may be enlisted when pain and terro become maladaptive.

The dream has been presented as a potential vehicle to capitalize upon this adaptive system. It is an indwelling theater that may display highly personalized "films" to elicit any imaginable hyperarousal state with appropriate neuroendocrine responses.

Such mock hyperstress situations could theoretically generate the euphoria, analgesia, and tranquillity necessary to the dreamer to better enable him or her to handle waking stress situations. When functioning adequately, the horrific dream images could be rendered amnesic while allowing the positive neuroendocrine responses to exert their salubrious effects. The Iroquois dream enactments and hyperarousal phases of ritual trance and possession states were presented as examples of therapeutic systems that operate in a similar manner.

It was pointed out that in many hyperarousal situations there is a sudden reversion to a hypoarousal state, which commonly occurs through the omnipotence maneuver. Again, this flip-over may occur spontaneously or may be fostered by the healer. The omnipotence maneuver is experienced at the affective level as a flooding with peace and faith, and at the cognitive level by a belief in supernatural intervention.

The neuroendocrine basis for the omnipotence maneuver (or even if there is such a basis) is not clear. It is possible that the hyperarousal response generates an increasing volume of protective neurohormones until a critical level is reached, which then forms a platform, as it were, for the emergence of the omnipotence maneuver—the sensation of "massive doses of vitamins in the veins," the fumes of the "boiling medicine rising to the brain," the white light that "envelopes and provides divine tranquillity," and so forth.

NOTE

1. This chapter deals largely with speculations about endorphins and *psychological* stress as they may relate to healing practices. The relationship between physical stress, particularly strenuous muscular activity, and endorphins and healing practices have been dealth with elsewhere (see Prince, 1982).

REFERENCES

Akil, H., Richardson, D. E., & Barchas, J. D. (1979). Pain control by focal brain stimulation in war: Relationship to enkaphalins and endorphins. In R. F. Beers & E. G. Bassett (Eds.), *Mechanisms of pain and analgesic compounds* (pp. 239-247). New York: Raven.

Appenzeller, O., Standefer, J., Appenzeller, J., & Atkinson, R. (1980). Neurology and endurance training: 5. Endorphins. *Neurology, 30,* 418-419.

Aserinsky, E., & Kleitman, N. (1953). Regularly occurring periods of eye mobility and concomitant phenomena during sleep. *Science, 118,* 273-274.

Belluzzi, J. D., & Stein, L. (1977). Enkephalin may mediate euphoria and drive-reduction reward. *Nature, 266,* 556-558.

Bourguignon, E. (1968). World distribution and patterns of possession states. In R. Prince (Ed.), *Trance and possession states.* Montreal: R. M. Bucke Society.

Broughton, R. J. (1968). Sleep disorders: Disorders or arousal? *Science, 159,* 1070-1078.

Carr, D. B., Bullen, B. A., & Skrinar, G. S. (1981). Physical conditioning facilitates the exercise-induced secretion of beta-endorphin and beta-lipotropin in women. *New England Journal of Medicine, 305,* 560-562.

Chapman, C. R., & Benedetti, C. (1977). Analgesia following transcutaneous electrical stimulation and its partial reversal by a narcotic antagonist. *Life Sciences, 21,* 1645-1648.

Cleghorn, R. A. (1979). Endorphins—Morphine-like peptides of the brain. *Canadian Journal of Psychiatry, 25,* 182-186.

Dehen, H., Willer, J. C., Boureau, F., & Cambier, J. (1977). Congenital insensitivity to pain and endogenous morphine-like substances. *Lancet, 2,* 293-294.

Dement, W. C., & Mitler, M. M. (1975). An overview of sleep research: Past, present and future. In D. A. Hamburg & H. Keith Brodie (Eds.), *American handbook of psychiatry* (Vol. 6; 2nd ed.). New York: Basic Books.

Dobkin de Rios, M. (1976). *The wilderness of mind: Sacred plants in cross-cultural perspective.* Beverly Hills, CA: Sage.

Frank, J. D. (1961). *Persuasion and healing.* Baltimore: Johns Hopkins University Press.

Freed, J. (1980, May 10). The making of a Moonie. *Today.*

Freud, S. (1953). Psychoanalytic notes upon an autobiographical account of a case of paranoia (Dementia Paranoides). In S. Freud, *Collected Papers* (Vol. 3). London: Hogarth.

Globus, G., & Shulman, R. (1963). *Considerations on affective response to motion pictures.* Report, Department of Psychiatry, Boston University School of Medicine.

Guillemin, R. (1978). Peptides in the brain: The new endocrinology of the neuron. *Science, 202,* 390-402.

Hughes, J. T., Smith, T. W., Kosterlitz, H. W., Fothergill, L. A., Morgan, B. A., & Morris, H. R. (1975). Identification of two related penta peptides from the brain with potent opiate antagonist activity. *Nature, 258,* 577-579.

James, W. (1902). *The varieties of religious experience.* New York: Longman.

Kiev, A. (Ed.). (1964). *Magic, faith and healing.* London: Free Press.

Koestler, A. (1954). *The invisible writing*. New York: Macmillan.
Kosterlitz, H. W., & Hughes, J. (1977). Peptides with morphine-like action in the brain. *British Journal of Psychiatry, 130,* 298-304.
Leacock, S., & Leacock, R. (1975). *Spirits of the deep: A study of an Afro-Brazilian cult.* Garden City, NY: Doubleday.
Lee, R. B. (1968). The sociology of !Kung Bushman trance performances. In R. Prince (Ed.), *Trance and possession states.* Montreal: R. M. Bucke Society.
Levi, L. (1972). Sympathoadrenomedullary responses to pleasant and unpleasant psychological stimuli, and sympathoadrenomedullary activity, diuresis and emotional reactions during visual stimulation in females and males. In L. Levi (Ed.), Stress and distress in response to psychosocial stimuli (supplement 528 to *Acta Medica Scandinavica,* 191).
Mayer, D. J., Price, D. D., & Raffi, A. (1977). Acupuncture analgesia in man reversed by the narcotic antagonist naloxone. *Brain Research, 121,* 368-372.
Messing, R. B., Jensen, R. A., Martinez, J. L., Spiehler, V. R., Vasquez, B. J., Soumireu-Mourat, B., Liang, K. C., & McGaugh, J. L. (1979). Naloxone enhancement of memory. *Behavioral and Neural Biology, 27,* 266-275.
Metraux, A. (1959). *Voodoo in Haiti.* London: Andre Deutsch.
Pert, A. (1981, September). The body's own tranquilizers. *Psychology Today,* p. 100.
Prince, R. H. (1964). Indigenous Yoruba psychiatry. In A. Kiev (Ed.), *Magic, faith and healing.* New York: Free Press.
Prince, R. H. (1968). Can the EEG be used in the study of possession states? In R. H. Prince (Ed.), *Trance and possession states.* Montreal: R. M. Bucke Society.
Prince, R. H. (1976). Psychotherapy as the manipulation of endogenous healing mechanisms: A transcultural survey. *Transcultural Psychiatric Research Review, 13,* 115-133.
Prince, R. H. (1979). Religious experience and psychosis. *Journal of Altered States of Consciousness, 5,* 167-181.
Prince, R. H. (1980). Variations in psychotherapeutic procedures. In H. C. Triandis & J. G. Draguns (Eds.), *Handbook of cross-cultural psychology: Vol. 6. Psychopathology.* Boston: Allyn & Bacon.
Prince, R. H. (1982). Shamans and endorphins: Hypotheses for a synthesis. *Ethos, 10,* 409-423.
Seitz, G. E. (1967). Epena, the intoxicating snuff powder of the Waika Indians and the Tucano medicine man Agostino. In D. H. Efron (Ed.), *Ethnopharmacologic search for psychoactive drugs.* Washington, D.C.: Government Printing Office.
Snyder, S. H. (1978). The opiate receptor and morphine-like peptides in the brain. *American Journal of Psychiatry, 135,* 645-653.
Stewart, K. (1969). Dream theory in Malaya. In C. T. Tart (Ed.), *Altered States of Consciousness.* New York: John Wiley.
Torrey, E. F. (1972). *The mind game.* New York: Emerson Hall.
Wallace, A.F.C. (1967). Dreams and the wishes of the soul: A type of psychoanalytic theory among the seventeenth century Iroquois. In J. Middleton (Ed.), *Magic, witchcraft, and curing.* New York: Natural History Press.
Wittkower, E. D. (1970). Trance and possession states. *International Journal of Social Psychiatry, 16,* 153-160.

4

COMPARATIVE ECOLOGICAL STUDIES OF THE SCHIZOPHRENIAS

G. ALLEN GERMAN

Scientific conceptions of schizophrenia have undergone a major revolution over the past twenty years. Not since the early years of this century, when the work of Kraepelin and Bleuler led, in different ways, to the development of the status of the disorder *as a disorder* has there been so much revision of ideas and development of new, and potentially fruitful, approaches to the conceptualization of this major mental illness. This revolution is an ongoing process, and its effects have not yet penetrated to all corners of the psychiatric and related professions; change in thought has been quiet and undramatic, based upon a steady accretion of information from wide-ranging and diverse research studies. That many of these studies have been carried out in geographically and ecologically "exotic" parts of the world has probably led them to have less impact than they might otherwise have had, although that situation is probably now changing.

In 1961, those who held to the Kraepelinian concept of schizophrenia viewed it, implicitly or explicitly, as a unitary disease entity. The influence of Koch was all pervasive; the etiology was thought to be a specific organic deficit that required only increased effort and increased refinement of technique (perhaps with a degree of serendipity) to be revealed; the symptoms and signs were specific and invariable; the course and outcome was one of inevitable deterioration leading to a vegetablelike end state. The viewpoint was reductionistic; clinical material that did not fulfill these clearly defined expectations were not examples of "true" schizophrenia. Thus "true" schizophrenia was given a special set of names—it was process, or nuclear, or hard-core schizophrenia. Clinical states that fulfilled the symptomatic criteria for schizophrenia, but not the supposed etiological and end-state criteria, were, to a large extent, unconsciously ignored or consigned to a limbo where the use of terms such as "psychogenic psychosis," "oneirophrenia," "schizophreniform psychosis," "pseudoneurotic schizophrenia," or "borderline states" demonstrates the confusion.

On the other hand, those who espoused the more Bleulerian view of the psychosis, leavening with a substantial bolus of Freud and a soupçon of Adolph Myer, were more flexible in their approach and more distinguished by their capacity to tolerate ambiguity. Most variants of human behavior might appropriately be labeled schizophrenia in their view, and in consequence a variety of treatments were found to be effective for "schizophrenia," the outcome was regarded as unpredictable, long-term psychotherapies worked, although later, when the funding basis for psychotherapy changed, it was demonstrated that short-term psychotherapies worked equally well. Patients who couldn't afford psychotherapy deteriorated in institutions and some charismatic operators persuaded the more gullible that schizophrenia was a myth.

In this confused situation the potential for change occurred with the dawning realization in the 1950s that psychiatrists in Britain and psychiatrists in the United States were not talking the same language when they talked of schizophrenia. The establishment of the Transatlantic Diagnostic Project during the 1960s, and its subsequent development, had a dramatic impact on thought about schizophrenia. It became increasingly accepted that theorizing about the nature of the disorder had to be put aside while an operational definition of what was meant by schizophrenia was hammered out. Symptomatic criteria for the diagnosis were developed, and clinical methods of establishing the presence or absence of symptoms were elaborated. These techniques were standardized in various assessment instruments such as the Present State Examination (PSE) and the Research Diagnostic Criteria. By utilizing these instruments, researchers and clinicians, at least in the United States and the United Kingdom, could begin to feel with some degree of certainty that when they talked of schizophrenia they were talking about the same thing. These developments represented a major breakthrough.

The essence of this development, it would seem, was that thinkers became prepared to say, "We do not know what this condition is so we will establish a convention for identifying people with similar symptoms and signs, and, having identified them, we will try and find out what is going on." This is the essence of the difference between the operational approach and the divine. The breakthrough, in psychiatry, was of the greatest significance; it marked a shift away from Aristotelian essentialism, with its expectation of finality and discovery of the essence, to a Socratic empiricism in which hypotheses are not confused with "facts" and where research is seen to lead to better explanatory hypotheses but never to final certainty. This shift away from essentialism (beliefs) to operational scientific enquiry should be stressed in a discussion of this type, since it is a shift that owes much to the development of cross-cultural studies in psychiatry, particularly as exemplified by the approach of the World Health Organization, and especially that approach as it has developed in relationship to the problem of schizophrenia. The change in approach ensures that current research strategies will increase knowledge in the behavioral sciences in a manner similar to that which has occurred in the natural sciences.

These philosophical and practical changes have altered our view of schizophrenia significantly. Particularly striking is the movement away from "single-mechanism" or "single-illness"-type formulations. In the area of etiology it is generally accepted now that multiple interacting factors operate. Thus the geneticists have shifted from simple Mendelian explanatory models to the view that inheritance in this disorder may be polygenic; while still looking for specific abnormalities, biologists increasingly conceptualize in terms of complex impairments of integration between hierarchical structures in the central nervous system; psychologists have ceased to suggest that schizophrenia is to be understood in terms of relatively simple behavioral deviations; and social scientists are less inclined to suppose that cultural differences are distributed in a simple bimodal manner as between developing and developed societies, or as between well-communicating families and ill-communicating families.

Nor is etiology alone now conceptualized in multidimensional terms: Clinicians have become increasingly willing to think of schizophrenia as the "schizophrenias" or as the "schizophrenic syndrome." Multidimensional as the etiology may be, it does not necessarily lead to the same pathological entity, with the same clinical picture and the same course and outcome. Tools such as the PSE, while permitting the identification of common symptom complexes with a fair degree of reliability, do not necessarily lead to the conclusion that these common symptom complexes reflect the presence of a single condition. These conceptual changes in the view of schizophrenia, while arrived at quietly, and while not as yet shared by all, have ushered in a new era in schizophrenia research characterized by the development of experimental studies and the evolution of hypotheses of greater heuristic value than previously. Some suggestive new information is already emerging, but the process of refining investigatory tools, and using these tools to expand the data base, are the more important characteristics of the present state of development.

CURRENT WESTERN CONCEPTS
OF SCHIZOPHRENIA

The Western concept of schizophrenia has therefore become a much more operational one, in which it is accepted that etiology is heterogenous and in most cases obscure. Similarly, it is accepted that the outcome is variable. The justification for using the term "schizophrenia" must rest on the presence of a modestly homogeneous clinical picture. Despite these advances in thought, problems persist.

First of all, there are situations in which the defined clinical picture of schizophrenia can be shown to be secondary to the occurrence of other illness or situations. Thus schizophrenic clinical pictures are not uncommon in the setting of manic or depressive disorders, particularly in adolescence; in the puerperium; in the presence of organic brain disease; as a result of drug abuse, particularly with amphetamines; in temporal lobe epilepsy; and in immediate response to acute and obviously related stress. These types of schizophrenic clinical pictures are variously referred to—as "schizophreniform psychosis" or as "reactive schizophrenia," or as "symptomatic schizophrenia." The latter term is preferred here as being consistent with usage in other branches of medicine.

While this separation of symptomatic schizophrenia may appear simple, in practice this is not always the case. In many circumstances the primary diagnosis is concealed, obscure, or not detected. This, to a degree, reflects the sophistication of investigation of each case of schizophrenia seen. The introduction of computerized axial tomography (CAT) in recent years has increased the number of cerebral pathologies detected in many cases of schizophrenia, thus moving these into the symptomatic group. Nevertheless, despite these difficulties, it seems desirable to separate these symptomatic schizophrenias from the remainder. They need not be excluded from research on schizophrenia, but should form a separate cohort, of great potential value as a comparison group alongside those schizophrenias where etiological precedents are obscure.

This latter group—the traditional mainstream nuclear or process schizophrenia—might be better referred to as "idiopathic schizophrenia," again a usage consistent with the pattern in other branches of medicine. Idiopathic schizophrenia was clearly regarded as a unitary disease up until the decade of the 1960s, but this notion has more recently become eroded. The ideas that such cases *always* had an insidious onset, a premorbidly schizoid personality, and were associated with a poor outcome have had to be dispensed with. In idiopathic schizophrenia a variety of onsets may be noted, and the outcomes appear to be variable. The situation is further complicated by those symptomatic cases where the effective treatment of the primary condition does not lead to resolution of the schizophrenic clinical picture, and where there is continuing deterioration as in some idiopathic thought disorders. Also, it is likely that in any group of schizophrenics thought to be idiopathic there may be a certain number of symptomatic cases undetected because of failure to detect the primary antecedents.

For these reasons, following the establishment of the presence of a schizophrenic picture, strenuous efforts must be made to exclude symptomatic cases from case material for research study. This is particularly so if research studies are conducted in various parts of the world on a comparative basis. Clearly, in many countries where standards of medical care are poorly develcped, there will be an excessive number of patients with schizophrenic symptoms that are secondary to physical disease, drug abuse, brain damage, and parasitic infestation. In some cases subnutrition in respect to vitamins and other essential foodstuffs may be relevant and in others acute cerebral disturbance superimposed on preexisting brain damage may be a possibility. The detection of such symptomatic cases may be very difficult given the unsophisticated investigative facilities available in many countries. Nevertheless, any international comparative study, if its results are to be useful, must grapple with this problem in developing a sound research methodology.

Returning to Western views of schizophrenia, it would be reasonable to say that the division of schizophrenia as between idiopathic (process, nuclear) schizophrenia and symptomatic (schizophreniform, schizoaffective, and so on) is in vogue at the present time. However, other approaches have been adopted, particularly by the

TABLE 4.1

Nomenclature and Diagnostic Criteria for Schizophrenia
and Schizophreniform Illness

	Good Prognosis	Poor Prognosis
Diagnostic terms		
	schizophreniform illness	schizophrenia
	acute schizophrenia	processs schizophrenia
	schizoaffective schizophrenia	nuclear schizophrenia
	reactive schizophrenia	chronic schizophrenia
	remitting schizophrenia	nonremitting schizophrenia
Diagnostic and prognostic criteria		
Mode of onset	acute	insidious
Precipitating events	frequently reported	usually not reported
Prepsychotic history	good	poor; frequent history of "schizoid" traits (aloofness, social isolation)
Confusion	often present	usually absent
Affective symptoms	often present and prominent	usually absent or minimal; affective responses usually "blunted" or "flat"
Marital status	usually married	often single, especially males
Family history of affective disorders	often present	may be present but less likely
Family history of schizophrenia	absent or rare	increased

SOURCE: From *Psychiatric Diagnosis,* second edition, by D. W. Goodwin and S. B. Guze. Copyright © 1974, 1979 by Oxford University Press. Reprinted by permission.

influential St. Louis School in the United States. Thus, in the textbook *Psychiatric Diagnosis* by Woodruff, Goodwin, and Guze (1974; see also Goodwin & Guze, 1979), an attempt is made to divide all schizophrenic clinical pictures into those with a likely good prognosis and those with a poor prognosis. The terminology, "good prognosis schizophrenia" and "poor prognosis schizophrenia," is suggested as being a reasonable terminology to use in referring to the whole spectrum of schizophrenic clinical pictures. Even this reasonable approach does not appear to solve the problem, as may be exemplified by Table 4.1, which is from *Psychiatric Diagnosis.*

With reference to this table, Woodruff et al. state that if the criteria for good prognosis schizophrenia are adhered to, the clinician will be correct 50 percent of the time—hardly an encouraging figure. On the other hand, the estimation of a poor prognosis, as based on the criteria for that prognosis listed in the table, will lead to a correct statement of prognosis 80 percent of the time. While this latter figure is somewhat better, it demonstrates that even where the clinician has sought to isolate what is essentially the idiopathic schizophrenic group, in at least 20 percent of these cases an unexpectedly good prognosis may eventuate.

Faced with these problems of varying etiology and varying outcome, it would appear that the most sensible approach is to first of all establish the presence or absence of a clinical picture of schizo-phrenia utilizing strictly defined inclusion and exclusion criteria; once this has been done, it is imperative to separate from the case material as many cases as possible where clear and relevant antecedents can be detected. On completion of these two steps one should expect to have a pool of largely idiopathic cases relatively uncontaminated with a variety of symptomatic reactions, together with a comparison group of symptomatic material.

Agreed-upon criteria for the establishment of the presence of a schizophrenic clinical picture are now available. These are probably best described in the *Diagnostic and Statistic Manual of the American Psychiatric Association* (DSM III), to which reference should be made. The DSM III definition is a purely operational one based upon symptoms and signs being present up to a certain required minimum. One of the interesting criteria added to DSM III is the requirement that symptoms have been present for at least six months. This has been criticized since it will increase the likelihood of more chronic cases being included in any group diagnosed as schizophrenic by DSM III criteria. Patients in whom there is an episode of characteristic schizophrenic clinical symptomatology, but whose illness has begun, run its course, and disappeared in less than six months will not be classified as schizophrenic using DSM III criteria. Nevertheless, the clear and straightforward statement of required criteria for diagnosis is a considerable step forward and enables comparative studies to be undertaken without so much likelihood that different groups will be observing different conditions.

In addition to these DSM III operational criteria for the diagnosis of schizophrenia, there is now widespread agreement that the presence of clear affective symptoms, either manic or depressive, is more likely to be associated with a future diagnosis of affective disorder, and a future course and response to treatment characteristic of affective disorder. In other words, the presence of clear-cut affective symptoms in the clinical picture should lead to a diagnosis of affective disorder, this condition taking precedence over schizophrenia in a diagnostic hierarchy. Similarly, should confusional symptoms be present, or other symptoms characteristic of established organic brain disease, then the diagnosis in the first instance should be organic brain disorder irrespective of the presence of affective symptoms or schizophrenic symptoms or both. In other words, prominent affective or confusional symptoms should categorize the case as "symptomatic."

While it is reasonable to see these defined characteristics as reflecting current Western concepts of schizophrenia, it is also important to point out that throughout the Western world many psychiatrists adhere to older methods of diagnosis and classification of the disorder, while others use idiosyncratic and personal systems for the definition of this condition. There continues, therefore, to be confusion, which is only likely to diminish as established systems of diagnosis, such as those of DSM III or of the PSE/CATEGO system become widely accepted in day-to-day clinical practice.

In summary, then, there is generally agreement as to the clinical picture necessary for the diagnosis of schizophrenia. Given the utilization of standardized diagnostic methods, and given the exclusion of symptomatic cases, it should now be possible through careful research to describe to what extent this clinical picture is associated with a variety of potential etiological variables and with a variety of outcomes. It is particularly important to make these observations in different cultures and in different ethnic groups in various parts of the world, for reasons that will be discussed in the next section.

THE CROSS-CULTURAL APPROACH

The term "cross-cultural" is one that has become sanctified by usage. However, the type of research it is still used to describe encompasses, or should encompass, more than just cultural variables. The title of this chapter indicates a preference for the term "comparative ecological" over "cross-cultural." Variations in the cultural matrix within which schizophrenia develops must be studied in detail, and the relationship of these variations to the mode of onset, the clinical characteristics, and the outcome of schizophrenia must be analyzed. However, if it is accepted that schizophrenia is a complex disturbance of biological, psychological, and sociological integration, then it follows that natural experiments that allow for variation in *all* these dimensions must be set up. *To date the main thrust of investigation of schizophrenia, as it is found in different geographical settings, has focused on differences in culture as between these settings.* Future research must include the other components of the matrix, because of the obvious fact that these diverse geographic settings are characterized by diversity of gene pool, biological development, physical environment, and ambient physical disease. These variables, together with social and cultural variables, interact and influence one another. To isolate aspects of each as independent variables is not an easy task, but it is one that must be addressed. The identification of diverse human ecological settings that permit one or another of these variables to be treated as the independent variable is an important task. The studies under discussion are, or should be, studies of diverse human ecologies and the relationship of *all* the characteristic features of these ecologies to the operationally defined symptom complex that is called schizophrenia.

Until all these factors are considered, even where research has been carefully planned and undertaken with rigorous and repeated checking, and the results have been analyzed adequately in a sophisticated way, no hypothesis can be generated that is other than one based on partial data. While all hypotheses should be regarded as interim, hypotheses based on partial data are really no more than suggestions. For example, it was a series of observations by Lambo during the late 1950s and the early 1960s on the apparently better prognosis of schizophrenia among preliterate Nigerians that led to the intense current interest in the variable prognosis of schizophrenia in different geographic settings (Lambo, 1960). In these studies Lambo suggested that only literate Nigerians showed a pattern similar to that found in Europeans and implied that cultural differences, as between preliterate and literate Nigerians, were responsible. However, it must also be recognized that the entire biological and physical environmental background of a literate Nigerian is probably very different from that of a preliterate Nigerian. Obstetrical care at

birth, nutrition, protection from disease, and stimulation of physiological and psychological development are all likely to have been
more adequate, or of higher quality, for the literate Nigerian than for
the preliterate.

These comments are not intended to reopen old wounds relating to
time-wasting and destructive controversies between nature and
nurture theorists. It is to be hoped that researchers have moved
beyond that stage. What *is* suggested is that a term such as "comparative ecology" better encompasses what should be the nature of these
basic researches in schizophrenia than does the term "cross-
cultural." Such usage might also persuade biologists concerned
about behavior to be more mobile in their research activities than they
have been in the past. While social scientists have always found
positive reasons for undertaking research in distant parts of the globe,
biologists have been much more laboratory bound, finding it difficult
to forsake their technicians and their technology for those places
where fungi grow on electronic components and the maintenance of
equipment is less readily guaranteed. Also, many psychiatrists tend
to view the word "cultural" as referring to esoteric aspects of their
discipline with which, as practical medical people, they need not
concern themselves. These strictures are not an attack on the cross-
cultural approach. It must be stressed that cross-cultural and social
studies have not only been necessary (and are necessary) but have
been fruitful, and are increasingly fruitful, in producing valuable
hypotheses and important new insights into schizophrenia. But it is
clear that the disciplinary base of these studies needs to be
broadened. In this respect one would agree with Edgerton (1980)
when he notes that psychiatric research in Africa has rarely been
multidisciplinary. However, while Edgerton is calling for the greater
involvement of social and cultural scientists rather than just psychiatrists, the plea here would be a somewhat different one. Certainly one
would wish to see well-trained social scientists deeply involved in
such studies, together with psychologists and epidemiologists. But it
is not true, as Edgerton suggests, that neurological, biochemical, and
genetic aspects of psychiatry are taken care of in the cross-cultural
setting by extensive use of psychiatrists. While psychiatrists are in
theory well-grounded in medicine, there are in fact very few psychiatrists capable of undertaking biological research at the level required.
One has to agree with Ellard (1979) that too often psychiatrists are "a
gaggle of untrained social workers who were once exposed to a
medical school."

SOME KEY FINDINGS IN
CROSS-CULTURAL RESEARCH

A comprehensive review of all the data that cross-cultural research has produced bearing on the problem of schizophrenia will not be undertaken here. That has been done adequately elsewhere (for example, see Jablensky & Sartorius, 1975; Day, 1980). It is important, however, to select some of the more significant output from these studies and to highlight why such output is significant.

First of all, studies coordinated by the World Health Organization (WHO) have established that tools can be devised for the reliable assessment of mental state phenomena across all sorts of differing cultures, even when these tools are used by psychiatrists of differing ethnicity, differing training backgrounds, and undoubtedly (psychiatrists being what they are) differing orientations to the discipline. Furthermore, it has proved possible to use these tools, with reliable results, in a variety of different languages. The Present State Examination (PSE) is the best known of these instruments and, in its various forms, the PSE can now be used reliably in any setting to identify, and to a degree to quantify, these symptoms and signs that are to be regarded, for the moment, as the necessary and essential data for a diagnosis of schizophrenia. Thus an essential variable—that is, the symptomatic basis of schizophrenia—can now be controlled. Apart from the PSE other instruments, designed to measure disability and social competence and to separate these from primary illness features, are in the process of evolution, testing, and usage. Other instruments are being evaluated and utilized that may prove capable of reliably identifying and measuring complex variables such as family attitudes to psychotic members (Sartorius, 1980; Jablensky, Schwarz, & Tomov, 1979). Apart from such notable developments there have been several secondary consequences of the deployment of these assessment instruments. Psychiatrists in many different centers have become aware of the importance of careful definition and observation in assessing mental state phenomena; they have learned the need for identical clinical techniques in the elicitation of abnormal signs—something that physicians have used for many decades, but that, in psychiatry, seemed to be an impossible objective only twenty years ago.

These are great achievements, but it would be wrong to note them without also noting certain potential hazards. It is of vital importance that it not come to be supposed that "schizophrenia" is now identifiable as an *entity* in terms of what the PSE and the associated CATEGO computer programs say it is. That would be to return to the earlier philosophy of essentialism. The PSE/CATEGO definition of schizophrenia should be regarded as an interim one only, to be constantly modified, shaped, and altered by data derived from research.

Another danger lies in the supposition that questionnaire-type instruments, however well standardized, validated, and deployed, are capable of measuring all the subtleties of complex variables such as those underlying cultural and individual attitudes. Edgerton's (1980) strictures are well made in this respect. Finally, the advantages of having such tools available as the PSE seem to lead some researchers and potential researchers to believe that to obtain reliable data, no more need be done that to obtain a PSE questionnaire and apply it to patients. The misuse of these instruments is a great danger, particularly when their proper use demands rigorous and uniform training with repeated retraining.

Second, the WHO collaborative studies of schizophrenia have produced results that clarify some aspects of psychiatric theory about the disorder. The international pilot study of schizophrenia (IPSS) has convincingly demonstrated the following:

(a) that the symptom complex that constitutes the disorder is present in all cultures so far studied; and
(b) that in all of these cultures schizophrenic disorders are to be found that have a benign course, a remitting course, and a malignant deteriorating course, although perhaps in different proportions.

There is no evidence that new varieties of schizophrenia have been detected, nor is there any evidence that varieties of schizophrenia previously described in more developed countries are absent in other parts of the world. These findings argue a fundamental and universal type of human response to some as yet unknown pathology or pathologies. They clearly demonstrate that schizophrenic disorder is not the exclusive property of certain types of society, of certain types of child-rearing practices, or of certain levels of economic development or educational development or technological development. If such factors are relevant to schizophrenia, their relevance must be in terms of influence rather than in terms of primary causation.

Third, these recent studies have demonstrated that in all the societies and cultures so far examined, the constellation of signs and symptoms designated as schizophrenic are regarded as morbid, both by traditional practitioners of medicine and by the general public. The reality of schizophrenia as an identifiable and pathological state is thereby confirmed. Its occurrence and course can no longer be supposed to be exclusively a consequence of "labeling," or of institutionalization (many schizophrenics in developing countries have never been institutionalized), or a result of scapegoating by a society that is alienated and unwittingly psychotic. Again, if such factors are relevant to schizophrenia, their relevance must be seen in terms of modifying influences rather than in terms of primary and necessary causes.

Fourth, the international pilot study of schizophrenia and the subsequent international study on the determinants of the outcome of schizophrenia have shown that traditional predictors of outcome are nowhere particularly reliable. Thus the five best predictors of outcome account for only a small proportion of the variance in outcome—a proportion that ranges from 8 percent to 22 percent across the different centers. For the fifteen best predictors of outcome taken together, these account for no more than 27 percent of the variance (Sartorius, Jablensky, & Shapiro, 1977). Nevertheless, these traditional predictors are somewhat more useful in developed countries (where they have evolved) than in less well-developed societies. Sartorius et al. (1977) conclude that these findings "suggest that no single factor and no combination of a small number of key factors have a very strong association with the course and outcome of schizophrenia and also that part of the variance in the course and outcome of schizophrenic patients . . . might be related to factors not included among the variables assessed." Whatever the cause of that part of the variance not accounted for, it is a very large proportion of the variance. These studies demonstrate that, even if they are not powerful predictors, factors such as social isolation, single life, a history of past psychiatric treatment, poor psychosexual adjustment, an unfavorable environment, a longer duration of the length of the target episode prior to initial evaluation, and flatness of affect are all associated with a poor outcome. If outcome can be predicted by relating it to identifiable premorbid and other factors, then it seems reasonable to conclude that while the wrong variables are not necessarily being looked at, a large number of very important influences on the course of this disorder have not yet been identified—or, alternatively, there has been failure to identify one or a few variables of massive influence.

Fifth, these studies suggest that the prognosis for schizophrenia is significantly better in developing societies than it is in developed societies. However, for a variety of reasons, mainly of a methodological sort, this can only be regarded as a suggestion at the present time, for reasons well discussed by Day (1980). Some of these problems include possible sampling errors (patients included in these studies were patients who *presented* at mental health facilities), a relatively low follow-up rate in the center that returned the best outcome profiles, and the possibility that varying outcomes might reflect varying proportions of different types of schizophrenia being present in different countries because of selective survival of those least predisposed to the disorder. This last assumes that the heavily predisposed, theoretically those likely to have the worst prognosis, might be biologicaly more vulnerable and at various stages suffer attrition by death. Nevertheless, the suggestion of better prognosis is there, and it is a suggestion that has been made by previous researchers (Murphy & Raman, 1971; Murphy & Taumoepeau, 1980).

These various studies all suggest that a single episode with a benign course is much more common in certain types of society or ecology. However, they do not always demonstrate that the proportion of bad prognosis schizophrenia is particularly low in certain societies. For example, in the study by Murphy and Raman (1971) based on the population of Mauritius, the proportion of Mauritian schizophrenics remaining severely disturbed at follow-up was greater than the equivalent proportion in Britain (36 percent at twelve years, compared to 28 percent at five years). Also, there is a study by Westermeyer (1980) that suggests that in a population of peasants in rural Laos, a very high proportion of a group of psychotics (the majority of whom were probably schizophrenics) continued over prolonged periods of time to show gross limitation of social functioning in a variety of key areas traditionally thought to be affected by chronic schizophrenia. Thus this question of variable outcome in different cultures demands further substantial efforts before clarification is likely. Some of the directions such efforts might take will be discussed later.

Finally, these WHO-coordinated cross-cultural studies permit certain conclusions to be drawn about the stability of a diagnosis of schizophrenia across cultures and about certain relationships between such a diagnosis and a diagnosis of affective psychosis. With regard to diagnostic stability, the PSE assessment—backed up by the CATEGO classification of diagnosis—showed, when administered at initial evaluation and again at two-year follow-up, a highly significant stability in the diagnosis of schizophrenia (72 percent in Washington, D.C., and 100 percent in London). If schizophrenic patients had subsequent psychotic episodes these were predominantly of the schizophrenic type. Nevertheless, in these studies, 17 percent of patients had subsequent affective episodes. Despite this, these results would appear to support the concept of the temporal consistency of schizophrenic symptomatology.

Apart from the positive outputs from the WHO research program in schizophrenia, it should be noted at this time that these studies *do not* answer certain questions about schizophrenia. Thus they do not show that schizophrenia has the same incidence and prevalence all over the world, despite the fact that this is frequently said. Indeed, the information bearing on this point is somewhat dated, and unreliable. The IPSS was not developed as an epidemiological study, and this is why the populations studied suffer from selection biases and may not in face be representative of schizophrenic populations in any of the several centers. Indeed, they almost certainly are not so representative. It is therefore still not possible to make authoritative statements about the prevalence and incidence of schizophrenia as a whole, nor about schizophrenia with differing outcomes, in different places around the world. What studies are available (Jablensky & Sartorius, 1975) show prevalence rates per thousand that vary quite widely from different places and countries (from 1.1 per thousand to 10.8 per thousand). These rates are gleaned from numerous studies carried out at different times by many different workers. There is no likelihood that diagnostic approaches and methods of sampling were identical between these various researches. Little reliability can be placed on such reports. It is important, therefore, that multicenter collaborative studies should address themselves to the issues of incidence and prevalance. It is significant to note that the present development of the "determinants of outcome" studies involves the examination of total first-contact cases in each of the defined areas.

This will provide much more reliable cross-center data as to incidence and prevalence, although first-contact sampling may still be criticized as potentially missing certain categories of patients.

CULTURAL CHANGE AND SCHIZOPHRENIA

The effect of cultural change on schizophrenia has been examined with conflicting results. Although Odegaard (1932), on the face of it, suggested that Norwegian migrants to the New World had an increased risk of developing schizophrenia, the results could also be examined in terms of selection of predisposed individuals for migration. On the other hand, in another Scandinavian study, Haavio-Mannila and Stenius (1974) showed a lower rate of schizophrenia among migrants than amongst those who did not choose to migrate. Similarly, while Lin Rin, Yeh, Hsu, and Chu (1969) found no increase in the rate of psychosis over a period of fifteen years of considerable social and cultural change in Taiwan, Torrey, Torrey, and Burton-Bradley (1974) have produced evidence that the rate of schizophrenia is increased in those populations in Papua New Guinea where exposure to Western styles of culture has taken place. Such variable findings are very hard to assess in any simple way. It is possible that they are related to differing proportions of different types of disorder in the samples studied as between various settings, but research methodologies and approaches have differed as well, and dissimilar methods have been used in the assessment of schizophrenia. Thus the Scandinavian concept of schizophrenia does not always include those schizophrenialike clinical pictures that are thought to be produced by psychogenic mechanisms—the so-called psychogenic psychoses. These contradictory findings can be assessed only if the analysis can be undertaken with certainty that methodologies and conventions have been identical. Again, the importance of utilizing agreed-upon and refined methodologies in a planned collaborative study across geographic areas is emphasized.

Many other studies of this type could be described. It is doubtful if any of them add significant data to those produced by the IPSS and related research. It is probably that it is only in the context of the IPSS that one can make the statement that reliable conclusions have been reached, and even the IPSS conclusions are limited in scope and must be hedged with certain reservations as noted above. This is not so much a fault of the IPSS strategy as it is a reflection of the fact that collaborative studies are still in their infancy and have not yet addressed the numerous and obvious questions that could probably be answered through comparative ecological research.

Of course, it may be the case that cultural change of a certain type in a certain region is associated with an apparent increase in the incidence of schizophrenia, while in other regions the incidence remains static or even falls. One would not have to look for highly complex scientific reasons to explain such a phenomenon. The incidence of schizophrenia may, after all, be related to fluctuating variables that have nothing to do with culture, or that have nothing to do with those aspects of culture that currently attract researchers. This last is an important point. The definition of culture is by no means simple, and there is certainly neither an agreed-upon definition nor an agreed-upon method of describing those featues of a given culture that are of critical importance.

This is a major scientific problem. To some extent cultural differences may be thought to be in the eye of the beholder. There may be less variation from place to place than certain social theorists suggest. Certainly there may be less variation in those cultural characteristics that might be critical for certain aspects of schizophrenia. This problem requires intensive and critical investigation, both in terms of new conceptions and in terms of research-based data. At the present time there is evidence of variance in the mode of onset, the symptomatology, the course, and the outcome, not only between different "cultural" settings, but within what appears to be the same cultural setting. The rough division of the IPSS centers as between the developing world and the developed world represents a gross oversimplification. What might be called "cultural chauvinism" is clearly operating in the identification, by Western theorists, of other cultures that are viewed as uniformly and homogeneously "developing," or "extended-family based," or "mythical-poetical," or "subsistence," or "preliterate," or "non-technological," to mention but a few of the labels that have been used to describe what seem to Western eyes to be common features of almost every community that is non-Western. On the other hand, if one tries to get away from this all-pervasive type of ethnocentricity, it is clear that human beings have much in common in terms of the things they value, the things that give them pleasure, the forms in which they express their dependency needs, the basic profiles of their personalities, and the fundamental behavioral patterns they exhibit. In the final analysis this commonality might prove to be of much greater importance than supposed differences.

Nevertheless, differences *are* important, particularly when these differences have been elucidated by rigorously undertaken research studies producing data that can be reasonably regarded as reliable and valid. But the importance of such differences lies in their demonstration, not so much in the various theories put forward to suggest they should be there. Theories tend to be shaped by fashions, in particular by fashions in thought characteristic of various scientific disciplines. It is fashionable in our introspective and self-critical Western culture to extol the virtues of the extended family and to deprecate the negative aspects of the nuclear family and of rampant individualism. Value judgments enter into such fashions and an awareness that the distribution of such values is largely arbitrary must be increasingly developed among critically minded social theorists. If this cannot be achieved, then science is back with essentialism—intuitively perceived values being mistaken for experimentally derived and demonstrated relationships.

To a degree, the present phase of WHO-administered collaborative studies—namely, the Determinants of Outcome Study—is addressing itself to some of the above-mentioned problems *in the cultural context*. Biological determinants are again largely neglected in the present program of work. Nevertheless, current studies are addressing themselves to a variety of social, cultural, and environmental variables. It is already clear that analysis of these variables, and their relationship to outcome, is pointing up substantial differences between individual centers, whether these be located in the developing world or otherwise. Indeed, one might be forgiven for concluding at the present time that critical variables that appear to have some influence on symptomatology and outcome might be as numerous and as varied as there are centers in the research program. There is still some reason to suppose that one of these critical variables is differences in the basic assessment of operationally defined schizophrenic symptoms and signs—despite training in the use of the PSE. It may be that retraining and reassessment of the reliability of psychiatrists' use of the PSE have not been sufficient to overcome the impact of local practices and trends in symptom assessment and diagnosis. This is a matter than must be looked at very carefully.

DIRECTIONS FOR CONTINUING
AND FUTURE RESEARCH

Incidence and Prevalence Studies

Having arrived at the point where reliable tools are available for the operational diagnosis of schizophrenia, given that these tools are properly used, and where a substantial number of fieldworkers have been trained to use them, it is now of importance to obtain data in respect to both the incidence and period prevalence of schizophrenia in various geographic areas. This is not merely a matter of academic interest. Without such baseline data it is impossible to assess the representativeness of any given cohort or to determine the precise proportion of the patient population falling into different course and outcome categories. Quite apart from that, it is only by means of careful and accurate assessments of incidence and prevalence that the extent of variations in the appearance rate of schizophrenia in different parts of the world can be established. Exhaustive searches for first-contact patients at various official and nonofficial agencies, in a defined area, will go a long way toward providing data regarding these matters. But it should be realized that it is probable that not all new schizophrenics, particularly those in whom the onset of the disorder is insidious (for example, those with the classical course of simple schizophrenia, where vagrancy may precede the development of more detectable symptoms and signs), will necessarily be captured by a network of helping agencies. This will be particularly probable in developing countries, where large numbers of psychotic persons adopt a vagrant lifestyle and are exceedingly mobile.

However obtained, such basic data should make it possible to establish several cohorts of schizophrenic subjects, representative of the local distribution of the disorder, which should then be followed up over a prolonged period of time. In establishing cohorts, at least one should contain reasonably uncontaminated examples of idiopathic schizophrenia. In addition, a sample of symptomatic cases, detected in the initial screening, will usefully form another cohort for comparative purposes in studying antecedents, onset, clinical picture, response to treatment, and outcome.

Follow-up, to be most rewarding in terms of information, must be planned with maximum attention to methods of minimizing the attrition rate of members of each cohort over time. Follow-up rates of 48 percent (IPSS, Nigeria) are not acceptable in terms of firm conclusions.

Cultural Problems

Much closer attention needs to be paid to what is meant by culture, and to those cultural differences that may be of significance. Techniques must be developed for measuring such variables, preferably in a quantitative manner, so that there can be certainty that they actually exist and to what degree. It seems essential that a panel of social scientists, with expertise in social and cultural areas, particularly with reference to mental health, should be set up. The nature of this area of scientific activity is such as to have produced a large number of emotionally held, idiosyncratic, and ethnocentric ideas. The selection of experts to constitute such a panel will not be an easy task, but priority does need to be given to selecting scientists who have shown a preference for reliable and valid scientific methodologies rather than to ideologically inspired social theories.

Biological Variables

There is also a need, and a fairly urgent one, to establish a similar task force of biological and medical scientists to advise on the most appropriate biological studies likely to provide information about the origins of schizophrenia and about those biological factors that influence its management, course, and outcome. Some areas of necessary biological study will be mentioned in the following paragraphs. The task force in cultural and biological areas should be supported by some form of linkage because it is vital that these differing groups of scientists have some understanding of the impact of the others' area, and have an opportunity to submit their ideas to the scrutiny of their opposite numbers. The ideal would be to have a panel of social scientists with some familiarity in respect to biological influences on social variables, and vice versa. The interaction of biology, physical environment, and culture is so close that any attempt to consider these broad areas in isolation (as currently tends to happen) will greatly handicap future efforts to comprehend important aspects of the problem of schizophrenia.

Single-Case Studies

Given that cohorts of patients are available for repeated and long-term study, and that potentially fruitful areas for measurement and study have been elaborated, there should also be attention given to the identification of single cases representative of different types of schizophrenia in terms of mode of onset, clinical picture, course, and outcome. Such single-case studies, pursued over time, with intense evaluation of variables, are perhaps just as important as the study of groups. This is particularly so with extreme variants—variants that may be common in one population, but rare in others. For example, Murphy and Taumoepeau (1980) have recently described a study of psychotic disorders in Tonga. In a population of about 2250 people on the island of 'Eua, during surveys in 1977 and 1979, the authors appear to have identified only one case of classical schizophrenia (with a chronic and deteriorating course) having onset as far back as 1950. Apart from the fact that the prevalence of schizophrenia in this community is reported to be low, the occurrence of one solitary case of bad prognosis schizophrenia demands careful attention. If the proposition of the authors is correct (to the effect that the stable, traditional, mutually supportive society of 'Eua protects against the occurrence of schizophrenia, particularly that with a bad prognosis), then it becomes all the more important to consider why one person, apparently a fairly typical representative of her culture, should be so uniquely afflicted. Familial and genetic studies of such a case would be of considerable value.

Prospective Studies

The Tongan case noted above exemplifies another major problem. Any attempt to analyze such unique data is handicapped by the retrospective nature of the observations. This is a considerable problem when it is necesssary that researchers try to elucidate those vital determinants of the patterns of schizophrenia that occur prior to the clinical onset of the disorder. In this context there is a need for the repeated establishment of prospective studies of children at risk for the development of schizophrenia, similar to the long-term prospective work currently being undertaken in Mauritius. Such projects must be established repeatedly because, with the passage of time, new techniques of measurement, related to variables newly conceived as being of significance, must be incorporated in the experimental protocol. Such studies, particularly if they are set up simultaneously in diverse social and cultural settings, utilizing the same techniques of measurement, might well prove to be the most rewarding of all. The structure that has already been created through the IPSS would seem to lend itself to the establishment of this type of research project in several different parts of the globe.

Specific Biological Areas

It would be generally accepted that biological factors have something to do with the etiology of what is called schizophrenia, and may have something to do with its response to treatment, its course, and its outcome. In most major centers of psychiatric research there are sophisticated programs dealing with a variety of biological aspects of these problems in one way or another. Many of these studies are exceedingly esoteric and complex and it would be inappropriate to suggest that these become part of an international research program based on comparative and collaborative research.

Nevertheless, there are significant biological factors that could and should be assessed in different geographic settings. Indeed, it could be argued that, to the extent that comparative ecological work fails to take account of these variables, such work is rendered much less persuasive than it might otherwise be. An example has been given with reference to Nigerian work that suggested that preliterate schizophrenics had a better prognosis than literate schizophrenics. It may be that another pertinent example is to be found in the contradictory findings of studies of cultural change and the frequency of schizophrenic disorder. In situations where culture is changing toward more "Western" types, it has been shown that there is an increase in the incidence of schizophrenia (Papua New Guinea), a decrease in the incidence of schizophrenia (Scandinavian studies on migration), and a static situation with regard to the incidence of schizophrenia (Taiwan). In these circumstances it must be asked whether or not some variable other than a cultural one is influencing these observations. While there is room for discussion as to the key social variables that might influence schizophrenia, the great attraction of studies using cultural *change* as the focus of attention is that cultural change collapses many variables and encompasses supposedly relevant social and cultural issues—at least the situation could be formulated that way. These contradictory results are therefore of some significance and need explanation. Furthermore, as previously noted, the influence of social variables (considered to be of importance in schizophrenia), insofar as they can be shown to determine the variance in course and outcome of the disorder, have to date proved capable of explaining only 27 percent of that variance. These considerations make urgent the search for other measurable influences that must be detected to permit a fuller picture to emerge.

Very few genetic studies have been undertaken on those populations of schizophrenics so far documented outside developed countries. It is important that such studies be initiated as soon as possible. In the first place, it is necessary to know if genetic findings obtained in developed parts of the world will be matched by those from quite different societies and in quite different gene pools. Quite apart from that, certain types of studies of heredity would be capable of shedding light on vexed issues, such as the possibility of selective nonsurvival of those heavily predisposed to schizophrenia. For example, it would be of considerable interest to collect a series of monovular twins on the basis of one of these twins having a demonstrated schizophrenic disorder. Examination of the identical-twin pair, while providing information about concordance rates in different ethnic groups and social settings, would also provide data (if suitably controlled) about the attrition rate (from death) among the twins of the probands. Studies of this sort, related to the broad field of heredity, should be developed.

Retrospective data may also be available in respect to perinatal events, episodes of infantile malnutrition, and other forms of cerebral insult sustained by those who have subsequently developed schizophrenia, especially perhaps symptomatic schizophrenia. However, such retrospective data, as noted above, is certainly unreliable, and likely to be even more unreliable in situations where adequate documentation of previous medical histories is not available. Here again, carefully planned prospective studies of conceptions at risk, following these through birth, infancy, and maturity, would be of great significance.

It is frequently stated that, quite apart from schizophrenia, clinical psychopathologies in many developing countries are characterized by an excess of uninhibited emotionality in which, in particular, excessive fear responses are not readily extinguished. There is some evidence to suggest that such affect-laden states are associated with a relatively good outcome in schizophrenia as well as in other conditions. Generally these emotional variables in clinical states have been attributed to cultural differences. However, biological studies may have some relevance to this observation. Thus the pig is an animal in which the growth spurt of the brain resembles that of humans, coming just before and just after birth. If pigs are deprived of either protein or calories between the third and eleventh weeks of life, in a manner just sufficient to keep their weight static, but are fed liberally thereafter, when six months old they show heightened emotionality compared to other pigs—snorting, squealing, and rushing about to a greater extent in strange surroundings—and are unable to extinguish unnecessary fear responses as readily as other pigs (Barnes, Moore, & Pond, 1970).

Such observations are of great interest—and may be relevant to observations on emotionality and personality in human populations. Subtle brain damage could well be germane to certain aspects of those clinical syndromes contained within the concept of schizophrenia. Indeed, such brain damage might conceivably alter the prognosis for good or ill. Catatonic phenomena have long been associated with a good prognosis for schizophrenia. Such phenomena seem to have been much more common in developed societies in the past. The IPSS and related studies have shown an excess of catatonic types of schizophrenia in Agra in India. A significant body of neurological and psychiatric opinion is persuaded that catatonic features are a manifestation of organic dysfunction of the central nervous system rather than specific to schizophrenia. Part of this view is that these organic dysfunctions associated with catatonia are also associated with poorer socioeconomic conditions and poorer conditions of general health. If there is any logic linking these ideas, there may be in this phenomenon of catatonia evidence for certain types of brain damage, related to poor environmental conditions, shaping a particular type of cerebral response characterized by catatonic clinical features and what appears to be a better prognosis—at least a better prognosis in terms of traditional indicators of deterioration. Severe undernutrition in rats has been shown to lead to slower maturation in the EEG, and it is of considerable interest that accompanying cerebral deficits are reported to affect more severely the phylogenetically younger parts of the brain (Mourek, Agrawel, Davis, & Himwich, 1970). Phylogenetically younger areas of the brain are often referred to as "higher centers" and are significantly associated with behavioral development and control. The possible relevance of such findings to the problem of schizophrenia is obvious—all the more so because Mundy-Castle (1970) has shown an excess of delayed EEG maturation in rural Ghanaians compared to urban Ghanaians and has attributed this difference to impaired physiological maturation resulting from adverse environmental circumstances and a variety of essential deprivations.

These studies emphasize malnutrition, an obvious variable to be considered when undertaking comparative research. Other environmental hazards potentially damaging to the central nervous system (and for that matter to the gene) are more numerous in developing countries than elsewhere. Many other features of the physical endowment and environment of peoples in various parts of the world could be pointed to as potentially relevant to the entire problem of schizophrenia, perhaps especially to the problem of "symptomatic" schizophrenia.

The unavoidable conclusion of these observations is that a properly founded cross-ecological assault on schizophrenia must, from the beginning, take account of biological variables, and as soon as possible must incorporate studies aimed at teasing out their influence from the influence of social and cultural factors. To date this has not been done adequately.

Undoubtedly, many types of biological study are complex and difficult to carry out, requiring highly trained human resources, people of a type who are not always willing to move to the research area, and who are not frequently found among indigenous professionals in developing countries. Furthermore, it is assumed that complex biological investigations, dependent on technology, are expensive and difficult to keep going because of the need for an extensive and sophisticated technological support structure. Finally, for reasons noted above, many such biological investigations must be prospective. It seems likely that several of these problems have been exaggerated. Certainly there is a need to increase efforts to ensure that indigenous professionals from developing countries are afforded the opportunity of sophisticated training in biological methods of research in the neurosciences; but there are also large numbers of skilled biological scientists in various parts of the world who would be more than willing to undertake research in various countries. To date many of these have felt that there would be no interest in funding such research, or that laboratory facilities would not be available for them.

Or many have just not been approached in terms of stimulating their interest in the needs of the comparative ecological field for their talents. Modern developments in technology have led to the availability of relatively small, inexpensive, and robust data-processing hardware and electronic instrumentation for sophisticated neurophysiological studies, including studies of the EEG and event-related cerebral potentials. These developments have greatly reduced the difficulties of using such equipment in tropical and adverse environments.

On the other hand, genetic studies are not so dependent on instrumentation and require approaches that in many ways are much more similar to the methods of social scientists and epidemiologists. That such studies have not been extensively undertaken in the developing world might suggest that the problem is somewhat more complex and is of the same nature as the reasons for the widespread use of the term "cross-cultural" rather than "comparative ecological." It may be pertinent that most social scientists, particularly sociologists and anthropologists, are by training (and almost by definition) pointed toward the comparative field as an essential laboratory for their basic research philosophy. This may explain their quite proper extensive involvement in comparative psychiatric research. On the other hand, the lack of a similar philosophical attitude among biological scientists may explain the infrequency with which such people consider the comparative field as one that requires their skills—at least as far as the field of mental health and disordered human behavior is concerned.

The ideal cultural-social-biological study is difficult to envisage. Indeed, such a comparative study might be better broken down into pieces that can be related to one another. However, it does seem essential at this stage that current programs should pay more attention to the biological area in a variety of ways. First of all, in defining cohorts of detected schizophrenic patients for study, there need to be somewhat more elaborate steps taken to document relevant physical disease. Grosser conditions may well be detectable on the basis of careful physical and neurological examination, supported by routine laboratory tests. However, there are many possible contaminating physical disorders that are relatively difficult to detect, such as various forms of epilepsy, various chronic infections and infes-tations, and various vitamin and other nutritional deficiencies. the proper assessment of these demands that collaborative research centers have the laboratory facilities to investigate each patient admitted to a cohort properly.

Electroencephalography must be carried out, as well as studies of immune responses (the most obvious here is the Widal, to exclude the more silent presentations of typhoid). It should also be possible to conduct vitamin deficiency studies, blood level assessments of drugs of abuse, and laboratory examinations of feces and urine for parasites. Quite apart from these sophisticated investigative requirements, simple indicators of physical disease such as the Erythrocyte Sedimentation Rate and even the diurnal temperature should not be neglected.

The determination of which biological assessments would give the maximum returns in terms of screening out symptomatic cases of the schizophrenic clinical picture should be considered by the previously proposed working group in the biological area. Selection of key biological variables should then be followed up by methods of monitoring the careful use of these in screening in the various collaborative centers.

Although more detailed attention to the above would assist in clarifying the numbers of symptomatic cases in the case material, nevertheless, there are many other biological variables that are difficult to assess retrospectively. An example of such would be subclinical brain damage, which may require highly sophisticated technology for its detection. Even here, however, counts of dominant EEG frequencies might be considered as a possible method of weeding out those persons most likely to be suffering from such background damage. It could be postulated that the use of such careful biological assessments might so reduce the remaining cohort of idiopathic schizophrenia in certain centers as to suggest that the bulk of schizophrenia cases seen in these centers are symptomatic. This might be particularly so in preliterate populations, where there is a higher expectation of physiological deprivation and disease. It may be speculated that predictors of outcome, taken from developed societies, would be found to be of much greater significance in predicting the outcome of the much diminished, but pure, cohort of idiopathic schizophrenia; it might also be found that the bulk of good prognosis cases were derived from the cohort of symptomatic schizophrenias; if the majority of these were preliterate, then the original observations of Lambo (previously noted) might be confirmed in a most interesting manner.

The establishment and the maintenance of studies of this type require dedicated research groups operating in various collaborative centers. Ideally, these research groups should be recruited from the indigenous scientists in each area in question. However, some leavening of international scientific expertise would help to ensure consistency of standards and of measurement, particularly in studies that would need to be maintained over lengthy periods of time. While such an undertaking might be costly, costs could be reduced if the number of collaborating centers was limited.

A problem as complex as the problem presented by schizophrenia, which appears to depend on the influence of genetic and environmental variables operating on several brain systems throughout many years of development is unlikely to be clarified by limited and restricted research approaches. Considerable expenditure in terms of money, training, and human resources will be essential if adequate research programs are likely to develop and produce reasonably clear answers to these complex problems. Quite apart from the possibility of clarifying some or all of the problems of schizophrenia, prospective research related to the development and functioning of human systems may well shed light on human development in general, and the occurrence of certain conditions—such as hyperkinesis, conduct disorders, and various personality disorders—in particular.

REFERENCES

American Psychiatric Association. (1981). *Diagnostic and statistical manual of mental disorders* (3rd ed.). Washington, DC: Author.

Barnes, R. H., Moore, A. U., & Pond, W. G. (1970). Behavioral abnormalities in young adult pigs caused by malnutrition in early life. *Journal of Nutrition, 100,* 149-155.

Cooper, J., & Sartorius, S. (1977). Cultural and temporal variations in schizophrenia: A speculation on the importance of industrialisation. *British Journal of Psychiatry, 130,* 50-55.

Day, R. (1980). *Research on the course and outcome of schizophrenia in traditional cultures: Some potential implications for psychiatry in the developing countries.* Geneva: Division of Mental Health, World Health Organization.

Edgerton, R. B. (1980). Traditional treatment for mental illness in Africa: A review. *Culture, Medicine and Psychiatry, 4,* 167-189.

Ellard, J. (1979). The future of psychiatry in Australia. *Australian and New Zealand Journal of Psychiatry, 13,* 43-49.

Goodwin, D. W. & Guze, S. B. (1979). *Psychiatric diagnosis* (2nd ed.). New York: Oxford University Press.

Haavio-Mannila, E., & Stenius, K. (1974). *Mental health problems and new ethnic minorities in Sweden* (Research Report 202). Helsinki: Institute of Sociology, University of Helsinki.

Hare, E., Price, J., & Slater, E. (1974). Mental disorder and season of birth. *British Journal of Psychiatry, 124,* 81-86.

Jablensky, A., & Sartorius, N. (1975). Culture and schizophrenia. *Psychological Medicine, 5,* 113-124.

Jablensky, A., Schwarz, R., & Tomov, T. (1979). *WHO collaborative study on impairments and disabilities associated with schizophrenic disorders.* Geneva: Division of Mental Health, World Health Organization.

Lambo, T. A. (1960). Further neuropsychiatric observations in Nigeria. *British Medical Journal, 2,* 1696-1704.

Lin, T. Rin, H. Yeh, E., Hsu, C., & Chu, H. (1969). Mental diseases in Taiwan, fifteen years later: A preliminary report. In W. Caudill & T. Lin (Eds.), *Mental health research in Asia and the Pacific* (pp. 66-91). Honolulu: East-West Center Press.

Mourek, J., Agrawel, H. C., Davis, J. M., & Himwich, W. A. (1970). The effects of short-term starvation on amino acid content in rat brain during ontogeny. *Brain Research, 19,* 229-273.

Mundy-Castle, A. C. (1970). Epilepsy and the electroencephalogram in Ghana. *African Journal of Medical Science, 1,* 221-236.

Murphy, H.B.M., & Raman, A. C. (1971). The chronicity of schizophrenia in indigenous tropical peoples. *British Journal of Psychiatry, 118, 489-497.*

Murphy, H.B.M., & Taumoepeau, B. M. (1980). Traditionalism in mental health in the South Pacific: A re-examination of an old hypothesis. Psychological Medicine, 10, 471-482.

Odegaard, O. (1932). Immigration and insanity: A study of mental disease among Norwegian-born population in Minnesota. *Acta Psychiatrica et Neurologica Scandinavica,* Supplement 4.

Sartorius, N. (1980). The research component of the W.H.O. Mental health programme. *Psychological Medicine, 10,* 175-185.

Sartorius, N., Jablensky, A., & Shapiro, R. (1977). Two-year follow-up of the patients included in the W.H.O. international pilot study of schizophrenia. *Psychological Medicine, 7,* 529-541.

Torrey, R. F., Torrey, B. B., & Burton-Bradley, B. G. (1974). The epidemiology of schizophrenia in Papua New Guinea. *American Journal of Psychiatry, 131,* 567-573.

Westermeyer, J. (1980). Psychosis in a peasant society: Social outcomes. *American Journal of Psychiatry, 137,* 1390-1394.

Woodruff, R. A., Goodwin, D. W., & Guze, S. B. (1974). *Psychiatric diagnosis.* New York: Oxford University Press.

5

TRANSCULTURAL INTERVIEWING AND HEALTH ASSESSMENT

MADELEINE LEININGER

During the past two decades, I have been actively involved in the identification, formulation, and clinical use of nursing and anthropological concepts across population groups representing diverse cultural backgrounds (Leininger, 1970b, 1978a, 1979, 1980; Morely, 1981). As a consequence, a body of transcultural nursing care knowledge has developed and is being used by nurses and other health personnel. The knowledge domains include transcultural theory, caring concepts, interview and assessment methods, and hypotheses regarding client care from diverse cultural backgrounds.

As this knowledge has developed, transcultural nursing has emerged as a formal area of study and practice in nursing. The desired goal of this subdiscipline is to generate and transmit knowledge so that the quality of care to clients of different cultural values, beliefs, and lifestyles will be improved.

As a founder and leader in the field of transcultural nursing since the mid-1950s, I find an obvious need to help nurses and other health care professionals become aware of different cultural groups to provide holistic care and to meet special needs of clients (Leininger, 1967, 1970b, 1978b). Until recently, most clients have not received culturally based assessments, care, or treatment. It was apparent that cultural conflicts and stresses existed between health care personnel and clients that could impede recovery or influence the quality of services rendered to clients of different cultural lifeways. Transcultural nursing was developed to remedy such inadequacies in health care services. Today, wherever culturally based care has been utilized, one can find differences in the quality of care rendered and in client satisfactions (Leininger, 1970b, 1973, 1978a, 1979, 1981b; Marsella & Pedersen, 1981).

Although it has been rewarding to launch a new discipline, there have been difficult hurdles: reformulating knowledge from anthropology and nursing into new modes of thinking and practice for nurses; shifting nurses' thinking from a *unicultural* to a *multicultural* frame of reference; and encouraging some entirely different ways of working with clients and cultural groups. Unquestionably, ethnocentrism with a heavy reliance of nurses upon Anglo-American (Caucasian) professional health knowledge has been a major hurdle to overcome. There has also been a need to deal with the fears, anxieties, and ambivalences of nurses as they consider the use of cultural values and beliefs that differ from their own values. Ethnocentrism, cultural blindness, and establishing new or different modes of interviewing clients and providing nursing care have been major problems. Incorporating transcultural nursing content into teaching and practice has required time, patience, and many creative strategies (Leininger, 1978a, 1981a).

Since I hold that caring is the central, unifying, and dominant focus of nursing, cross-cultural caring values had to be identified, formulated, and incorporated into nursing curricula and practice settings (Leininger, 1981b). This emphasis has led to the identification of differential caring constructs that fit a designated cultural group's values and general health or caring lifestyle. Different caring values based on ethnographic research data have opened the door to a new approach to nursing and have stimulated new lines of transcultural nursing and health research. Transcultural nurse researchers and graduate nursing students have provided new lines of thinking and care practice based upon the identification of cultural care values.

The purpose of this chapter is to present some selected transcultural concepts, models, and guidelines related to interviewing, assessing, and measuring clients' responses or behavior modes from different cultures. The content is presented with the recognition that the body of transcultural nursing knowledge is still evolving with new knowledge and refinements based on research and clinical-field practices. Experiences and viewpoints from anthropology and other disciplines have been highly valuable in perfecting and knowing transcultural health and caring in their fullest dimensions. This chapter is, therefore, presented with the intent to share current transcultural nursing insights and to discover common knowledge domains useful to all health professionals, as well as to identify knowledge domains fairly unique to a particular discipline. Most important, mental health professionals across many disciplines appear ready to share knowledge and learn together in order to develop some entirely new approaches to mental health derived from cross-cultural theories, research findings, and therapy practices. I view this as an encouraging and promising new direction for psychiatric mental health professionals.

Detailed definitions of the concepts being used in this chapter are included in the Appendix.

RATIONAL FOR INTERCULTURAL INTERVIEWS AND HEALTH ASSESSMENTS

More and more people from different places in the world are interacting with one another. Understanding people with different cultural backgrounds has become a major problem for many people in our society and in the world. New modes of communication and rapid transportation are affecting our lifeways within and between cultures of different values. These trends will continue; they remind us that we are truly living in a multicultural world.

For health personnel who are expected to work with people of diverse cultures, the critical essential challenge is to discover ways to assess, communicate, know, understand, and work with clients effectively. Health personnel in the field of mental health are becoming aware of the importance of culture in diagnosis, assessment, and therapy (Draguns, 1979; Leininger, 1969, 1970a, 1970b, 1973; Marsella, 1979). Interviewing and assessing the cultural lifestyle of a client is a major and new challenge for most mental health personnel. It is an area requiring a much broader perspective of human behavior, and one that goes beyond an individual focus to group cultural behaviors, cultural systems, language systems, institutional values and norms, and diverse environmental forces. These are broad and comprehensive knowledge domains for which most mental health personnel have not been prepared in their educational programs. Nonetheless, they are critical and essential dimensions requiring urgent attention for mental health faculty, students, clinicians, and researchers. Focus on the inclusion of culturological data will provide some entirely new assessment and therapy modes for mental health personnel.

Another reason that cultural interviews and assessments are necessary is the desire of professional counselors and therapists to be effective, relevant, and successful in their work. If therapists are finding difficulty in obtaining clients and/or maintaining client contact, they will want to consider the role of culture in client services. Already many perceptive therapists in the mental health field are asking questions such as: How do I interview a client from another culture? How do I reach the client in an interview to know and understand the client's world view or concerns? What background knowledge do I need to make valid assessments and judgments about the client? How do I measure what I hear, see, and experience in an interview? How can I utilize the content gleaned from an interview for therapy or counseling purposes? Such questions and others point to the need for developing knowledge and skills in cross-cultural interviews and assessment modes.

Still another reason for culturologically based interviews and assessments is to change *unicultural* modes of viewing clients to *multicultural* frames of reference. The unicultural view that all clients are alike or partake of the same cultural lifeway is a myth. Client populations tend to be multicultural, and therefore health personnel need to consider a multicultural approach to interview, assess, and provide therapy. Mental health personnel must change to a multicultural mode of thinking and acting to meet their client, family, and population needs.

Culturologically based interviews and assessments are also needed to prevent cultural imposition and unnecessary cultural stresses and conflicts (Leininger, 1970b, 1976, 1978a, 1979; Spradley, 1982). Currently, one can observe many situations in which physicians, nurses, social workers, and others are unintentionally or intentionally imposing their professional values on clients. Unrecognized cultural conflicts, stresses, and tension states may place a heavy burden upon the client who is struggling to attain or maintain health. The imposition of one's professional and personal values on the client has ethical implications; this is a situation that needs far more attention than it is receiving to date (Leininger, 1979; Marsella & Pedersen, 1981).

The therapist who uses culturally based knowledge in interviews, assessments, and therapy can prevent the occurrence of unnecessary cultural conflicts and stresses. A culturally oriented interviewer and therapist will be able to value, use, and promote cultural accommodation, preservation, and repatterning according to the needs of the client. Such an approach is encouraging to a client who has never had this consideration with a unicultural or a medical model that focused primarily on symptom-disease interviews and physiologically based therapy. Client satisfactions and recovery outcomes tend to increase when cultural lifeways and values of the client are taken into full consideration in interviews and used in therapy (Leininger, 1970a, 1973, 1979). It is encouraging to see culturally oriented therapists preserve and maintain cultural values rather than demean, drastically change, or inadvertently ridicule them.

Most important, mental health therapists can gain new insights about their own cultural values and lifeways and how to manage their ethnocentric and related cultural threats to the client. Such a growth-promoting experience for mental health therapists or counselors is another major and largely unknown benefit gained from the use of culturologically based knowledge and interviews. Getting into the world of the client (the "emic," or local, view) and understanding the client's world view, values, and referent groups can provide many new insights for professional growth about self and others. From such experiences, I have repeatedly found health personnel greatly expanding their personal views of different cultures; they become more perceptive, sensitive, and receptive to diverse beliefs and lifeways. This makes them more effective therapists and more humanistically oriented people.

Last, but not least, culturological interviews and assessments tend to promote new lines of systematic inquiry with different theoretical postures and research methods. Cultural differences and variations within and between clients stimulate new kinds of research questions, problems, and theories. Comparative insights about human deviations, life problems, and struggling to maintain oneself are a few of the areas to be described, explained, or predicted. A variety of theories with testable hypotheses are emerging from interviews with clients or families of different cultures and leading to new and major theories about health diversity and universality of human behavior (Leininger, 1982).

THEORIZING AND CONCEPTUALIZING
AN INTERCULTURAL INTERVIEW

Before conducting a culturological interview to assess the health or illness status of an individual, family, or social or cultural group, the interviewer should conceptualize the multifaceted world of the interviewee. Multiple internal and external forces influence human behavior, such as world view, language, cultural values and lifeways, environment, and social structure features. To grasp the world view of the client or interviewee, a broad and holistic anthropological perspective is needed that includes knowledge about the client's cultural background or life orientation. How to help the interviewer think about and recognize multiple types of world forces influencing the interviewee's behavior—such as religious, kinship, political, and economic factors—is "mind stretching," or a different approach for the interviewer. Such knowledge is, however, important in gaining a holistic view of the interviewee and in determining the therapy goals and approach.

Traditionally, health care providers, counselors, and therapists tend to use a narrow view of a client (for example, the biological, physical, and emotional manifestations, or the internal forces affecting an individual). With a culturological interview, one thinks very broadly about the universe in which the client lives with a cultural group, and within a particular environment. Social structue forces (political, economic, educational, and cultural values, kinship and social ties) influence how the client knows and relates to people within or outside the health care provider's world. At the same time, there are particular internal body forces of the client that must be considered in relation to the broad world or external view of the client. But to shift the interviewer's thinking from the narrow cellular, or biopsychological, body-mind focus to consider social structure, cultural values, and behavior lifestyles is a very comprehensive apporach for most health professionals. The following theoretical statements are offered concerning this broad holistic framework:

(1) The more an interviewer is able to conceptualize, comprehend, and use world view, culture values, and social structure data influencing the client's behavior, the greater the evidence of a holistic viewpoint being used with the client.

(2) The greater the evidence that the interviewer possesses knowledge about the cultural beliefs, values, and general lifeways of the interviewee before the interview, the greater will be the signs of mutual satisfaction with the interviewer and interviewee.

(3) The world view, social structure, and cultural values and beliefs of the interviewer and interviewee are generally different; however, the more the interviewer actively listens to and creatively responds to the

interviewee's cultural data, the more signs of satisfaction will be evident with the interviewee.

(4) The greater the signs that the folk and professional health subsystems are different between the interviewer and interviewee, the more the signs of stress will be manifest in the interview.

Such theoretical statements help one think broadly about human behavior, and especially for a holistic perspective. I contend that this view is essential if one is to obtain an accurate and reliable picture of the interviewee.

As an aid in the attainment of the above goals (that is, a culturological interview approach), the Sunrise Model (Figure 5.1) is offered. The Sunrise Model was developed to assist health personnel to expand their thinking in order to enter and grasp the broad world view of the interviewee, client, or patient. This model has proved valuable to nurses, physicians, and others in their efforts to conceptualize the multiple and diverse components that influence client, family, cultural group, or community health-illness behavior. The prevention of illness and the maintenance of health patterns of clients can often be identified by health personnel if they regularly and systematically use the model to assess clients' needs or conditions. Students often say that this model stretches their minds to go beyond a traditional view of individual clients as biological organisms with diseases to human beings living in a large world with many factors influencing their behavior. The "sunrise" term aptly conveys the idea of a "new dawn" in health assessment and of the need to expand one's thinking to cultural factors.

In examining the Sunrise Model, one can identify several components (the world view, culture, language, environment, social structure, and folk-professional) influencing the client. Since every human being is born and lives in a particular world, these social structure components should be considered as critical and dominant forces influencing the health status and general lifeway of a client. Within the broad social structure, environment, world view, and cultural framework are the specific and diverse components of the social structure, namely, the technological, religious, kinship, cultural, political (legal), economic, and educational systems. These systems influence and give rise to the values and nature of health-illness systems in any society. Individuals, families, and cultural groups reflect aspects of these societal and environmental forces when they

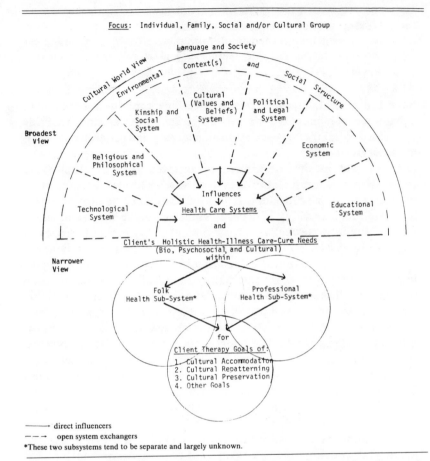

Figure 5.1   Sunrise Conceptual Model for Culturological Interviews, Assessments, and Therapy Goals

seek health care from professional personnel. Hence cultural values and social structure variables must be considered in an interview with an individual or family, and with thought as to how these variables affect the client's health and illness state. For example, an Amish family's religious system is a dominant force in health care assessment, and the client will endeavor to preserve his or her beliefs. In contrast, an Anglo-American white middle-class family tends to focus upon technological material and economical systems in trying to deal with losses and gains. The Gadsup of New Guinea focus mainly on kinship patterns and their relationship to health and illness.

Cultures vary with their emphases on each system of the social structure, which provides clues for health care services. The interviewer who listens and is knowledgeable about such variations will note these themes during the interview, and will explicate ideas that concern the client for therapy implications.

In eliciting data during the interview on these various factors, the interviewee's language and nonverbal communication must be considered thoughtfully. Clients from different cultures will use different body language or nonverbal expressions (Cole & Scribner, 1973; Leininger, 1976). Both verbal and nonverbal communication are important in assessment during the interview and in validating the meaning when possible. Body language expressions and vocal pitches in tone and intensity can help the interviewer grasp the feeling and importance of different aspects of the social structure elements of the interviewee.

In using the Sunrise Model, keep in mind that the individual, family, or social or cultural group should be *active participants* in the interview, with the interviewer. By keeping the interviewee as a *participant*, it makes him or her (or the family or social group) feel valued, important, and a partner in the interview process—sharing ideas that are important to the interviewee. The participant role of the interviewee greatly increases cooperation and facilitates a productive and qualitatively rich interview. As an equal participant in the exchange, the interviewee (especially one from a culture strange to the interviewer) often feels it is acceptable to share cultural ideas and to have them respected by the interviewer. If the interviewee is treated as a true participant rather than as "a person acted upon," he or she tends to share more detailed cultural data and will show signs of being trusted. If viewed as a nonparticipant or as a passive client, the interviewee generally perceives a status and role difference that limits or curtails the flow of content during the interview.

Turning to the lower part of the Sunrise Model, the folk and professional subsystems are quite separate worlds in this society and in other places in the world, and so the interviewer will need to learn about each subsystem. Knowledge of the client's cultural folk system will help the interviewer to learn about folk caretakers and curers (or healers) who have special roles and healing skills. There are also general differences between the folk and professional care-cure subsystems, which I have identified and discussed in another publication (Leininger, 1981c). The reader is, therefore, encouraged to study some of the dominant differences between these two worlds before initiating interviews, making clinical assessments, or conducting therapy with clients. If professional health interviewers are not aware of the folk subsystem, they may miss important information for assessment of the client's culturological behavior and health values or practices. Currently, some health professionals tend to deny the existence of a folk subsystem and may overtly demean or devalue folk ideas. It is anticipated that, in time, the folk and professional care-cure worlds will be more fully known and will be used routinely to help the client, and will be more valued in therapy or caring practices.

Using a holistic approach (that is, the client's biopsychosocial and cultural aspects, the interviewer elicits and assesses the folk and professional health subsystems in relation to content domains on the upper part of Figure 5.1 (broad social structure features, and so on) and determines the client's therapy goals. It is my theory that these therapy or assistive goals in the classificatory areas of cultural accommodation, repatterning, and perservation. However, other goals may be identified in the future.

The Sunrise Model is, therefore, a conceptual guide or cognitive map to help the interviewer (and often the interviewee) share ideas about the cultural world view of the interviewee. It is a model to help the interviewer (and therapist) assess the multiple variables influencing the interviewee to obtain a comprehensive, accurate, and reliable picture of the client as a basis for therapy goals. the interviewer uses this guide by focusing on major domains of inquiry or the broad cultural variables to elicit and study responses. From the interview, the interviewee's responses and patterns of behavior are identified and analyzed for cultural themes. Verbatim statements, specific life experiences, nonverbal expressions, and material cultural items carried or found with the interviewee provide the interviewer information about the client's world view and experiences. Focusing on multiple aspects of the interviewee's world requires the interviewer to handle large amounts of cognitive content and to synthesize and analyze themes of behavior. As the interviewer gains more experience with culturological interviews and assessments based on the Sunrise Model, his or her skills and cognitive synthesis abilities will increase.

In summary, the Sunrise Model has these major features:

(1) It is one of the most comprehensive and holistic-focused models in the health field to identify, assess, and learn about the multiple

culturological forces influencing individual, family, social, and cultural group behavior within a societal and world view perspective.

(2) It can help the interviewer to understand and value the role of culture, language, social structure, and environment upon human behavior, life experiences, and health status.

(3) It provides a conceptual framework to link broad features of a culture and society with narrower features related to individual and group health-illness behaviors to grasp the world view of clients.

(4) The model can be used by the interviewer at any place comfortable to him or her or the interviewee, that is, in the professional health subsystem or in a political, religious, or other type of context.

(5) The interviewee is considered an active and equal participant in the interview with respect to social structure, health (folk and professional), environmental, and general lifeways of the client.

(6) Comparative research studies can be done with respect to social structure and cultural variables with individuals, families and cultures as the variables are made in the model and can be used by other interviewers for comparisons.

(7) Data from the different aspects of the model tend to generate new or different theories, research designs, or different ways to help clients or establish therapy goals.

(8) The model can lead to multidisciplinary therapy and research according to different fields of knowledge and areas of expertise.

PRINCIPLES AND GUIDELINES FOR CONDUCTING A CULTUROLOGICAL INTERVIEW

The interviewer can prepare him- or herself to conduct a culturological interview by taking some cross-cultural courses or programs of study in anthropology, health nursing, sociology, biocultural studies, psychology, and ecology. In general, the interviewer should have a broad knowledge base about diverse culture, with their different values and lifestyles. Knowledge of the social structure systems, folk and professional health subsystems, cultural values, language modes, environmental factors, comparative behavior, and biophysical aspects will help assure a successful interview and health assessment. The use of anthropology films and direct contacts with cultures are other ways to increase the interviewer's knowledge base.

Initially, the interviewer should encourage the interviewee to share ideas and generally lead the interview exchange. The interviewer might introduce a broad subject area for discussion with statements such as the following: "I am interested in learning about some of your folk or home remedies and how you believe they help you to remain well." "Tell me about your folk practices." "I would like to learn about a typical day or night in your life." These are "grand tour" questions, but they permit the interviewee some latitude to talk about areas of interest to him or her. If the questions are tightly structured and many in number, this may curtail the interviewee's discussion of his or her world, and the questions may miss what is culturally relevant. Other interview techniques are discussed below.

The interviewer should be prepared to have three interview sessions of approximately 30-35 minutes in duration. Past and present interviews should be considered together, so the interviewee can continue with life experiences related to areas of the Sunrise Model. The first interview generally provides an introduction to the interviewee's world, whereas subsequent interviews provide in-depth knowledge about the social structure, values, and health-illness aspects, and validate ideas previously discussed. Psychologically, the interviewee generally finds the three-phase culturological interview more comfortable, acceptable, and realistic than one lengthier interview, with a trusting relationship developing with each interview. The interviewer may interview one person, a family, or a large group; however, it is best to start with one client until one gains more confidence and skill in handling cultural data.

The interviewer should expect to listen to individuals and families whose lives are linked with different cultural groups by marriage and life experiences. Personal prejudices and biased attitudes toward any particular cultural group should be assessed to prevent unnecessary conflicts and stresses during the interview. Cultural-awareness or sensitivity sessions may be available to help the interviewer with prejudices and ethnocentrism.

Finally, the interviewer should be aware of differences between a culturological or physical diagnostic (or assessment) interview. Consider the following differential points. First, a culturological interview focuses upon *themes and patterns of cultural behavior, healthy lifestyles, and environmental conditions in reference to the interviewee's familiar lifeways.* This contrasts with a psychophysiological interview, which often focuses on symptoms, diseases, and pathological medical conditions with a hospital, clinic, or professional environment.

Second, a culturological interview is a very broad holistic approach focusing on multiple societal variables that can influence health and illness lifestyles, whereas a psychophysical interview tends to focus on partial systems, organs, symptoms, and selected behavior features related to health-illness.

Third, the culturological interviewer uses an open-ended, relatively unstructured, and flexible mode of inquiry with the interviewee, permitting the interviewee to share ideas and experiences. In contrast, a psychophysiological interview focuses upon specific lines of inquiry and questions that are usually highly structured and closed-ended, requiring single-answer responses.

Fourth, the culturological interview is based upon *participant-observation* and *comparative* data, whereas the psychophysical interview relies more on the interviewee's specific response data to questions, or on specific illness conditions.

Fifth, a culturological interview relies more on a *"nontouch" approach* (but not completely) to the client, whereas physiological interviews are generally "hands-on," involving touching the client and the use of many different technological tools or equipment.

Sixth, the culturological interview gives more emphasis to *external* factors than to internal ones, whereas a psychophysiological interview tends to focus on internal body and immediate person-to-person experience factors.

Interview and Assessment

The following guidelines and principles are offered to assist an interviewer or to help the therapist conduct a culturological interview:

(1) *When feasible, conduct the interview in the individual's natural setting, such as his or her home or workplace, to get direct "eyeball"-validated data through firsthand observations and experiences.*

The primary reasons for this principle are to make the client feel "at home" or comfortable in his or her natural environment with his or her symbolic referents, and to validate the environmental context of interviewee statements. The interviewee's natural environment (that is, home, school, store, or the like) often stimulates ideas related to his or her cultural lifeways. Material objects are often stimuli for discussion and provide an inside view of the interviewee's world. Interviews in familiar or natural settings tend to elicit many ideas that can be documented *in situ*. Symbolic and referent meanings come alive when familiar settings serve as referents. Contextual meanings help the interviewer to understand many ideas associated with an object, event, or ritual ceremony. Granted, not all interviews may occur in natural contexts, but they are strongly recommended for the reasons just cited.

(2) *At the beginning, identify yourself, the nature and focus of the interview, and the general areas of interest or plans for the interview.*

It is essential that you inform the interviewee who you are and what your interview interests and plans are. For example, one might say, "I am Ms. Doe and I would like to talk with you about your lifeways and your cultural background. I am interested in learning about your daily activities or patterns of living. I would like to use this information to help me understand you so I can find ways to assist you." At the outset, discuss your plan to meet for three interviews of approximately thirty minutes each and of the general areas you wish to talk about. I also add: "I hope you will be comfortable to share as openly and candidly as possible about your lifeways so I can understand you—your beliefs, values, and forces that tend to influence your lifeway or health." Allow interviewees to ask questions of you and to clarify your comments or theirs.

(3) *Use the interviewee's native language. If this is not possible, then you should use a reliable interpreter.*

If the interviewer can speak the interviewee's language, this makes the latter more comfortable and increases the flow of communication. If an interpreter is used, identify and discuss key language words or statements that may be used before the interview session begins. The interviewer should know some frequently used words or phrases of the interviewee in order to be able to follow his or her ideas and to be sure the interpreter is sharing full and accurate data.

During the interview, remain alert to the interviewee's body language and voice inflections. Knowing a few linguistic terms often helps. Be sure you get accurate translations of the interviewee's statements and their meaning by occasionally rechecking ambiguous terms or ideas. The emic approach, which seeks local or native meanings, is recommended (Leininger, 1970b, 1978b).

(4) *Use a small pad to record a few key words or phrases as well as nonverbal observations.*

The use of a small pad (rather than large pieces of paper) helps prevent distractions during the interview. It also helps the interviewer focus on the interviewee and listen attentively to him or her, as well as observe body language and environmental clues. Excessive note taking or a tape recorder tends to reduce the flow of ideas between the interviewee and interviewer, and distracts the former from sharing ideas. Often attention to writing increases anxiety and arouses distrust in the interviewee. the interviewer mainly records on the small pad some key ideas, sequence of subject areas, and a few cue observations. *Immediately after* the interview, the interviewer writes out in full the cues recorded on the pad, describing incidents, identifying major themes of each content domain, and giving a generally full account of what the interviewee and interviewer said and did during the session. It is imperative to record the interview while ideas and experiences are fresh in one's mind to increase the validity of the interview. If you use a tape recorder, camera, and other devices, you need to clarify to the interviewee how you plan to use them. The notes are used to refresh one's memory before the next session and as primary source data for helping the client.

(5) *Interview in an open, friendly, respectful, and interested manner.*

Throughout the interview, it is important for the interviewer to maintain an open, friendly, and receptive attitude to the interviewee's comments. Show active and genuine interest in the interviewee's ideas or nonverbal signs. A nonjudgmental and noncritical posture about the interviewee's lifeways, beliefs, and values enables the interviewee to "tell it as it is" and not be frightened by the interviewer's appraisal of them. Remaining relaxed, calm, and friendly during the interview helps to maintain a favorable flow of ideas.

(6) *Throughout the interview, maintain an active listening and observing role with the interviewee, and a reflective attitute about what is presented.*

This principle is extremely important and is probably the key to a successful and effective culturological interview. Interviews by professional strangers and those whose culture is markedly different from that of the interviewee's are often stressful to both the interviewee and interviewer. When the interviewer is an active listener and observer as well as reflective about what is said or observed generally, it makes the interviewee feel his or her ideas and presence are important. The interviewer should listen to what is described of folk legends or about how things came to be valued and practiced. Observing the interviewee's body language (positioning) and other nonverbal communication modes may provide many ideas about the interviewee. For example, an Afro-American interviewee twisted two buttons off her coat as she talked about her views of being suppressed by political and legal leaders in the community. Another interviewee demonstrated the use of folk treatments by massaging her arm in a certain way. If the interviewee finds him- or herself discussing a stressful topic, the interviewer should not encourage changing the client topic unless the interview wishes to do so. The interviewer generally will find nonverbal body stresses associated with stresses, conflicts, and problems related to cultural changes.

(7) *Maintain a learning attitude; learn from the interviewee and do not assume to be the professional "expert."*

This principle is difficult for many professionals, who tend to remain experts or to know all the answers about people living. Since most professionals have limited knowledge about cultural values, meanings of cultural behavior, and material referents, they should try to be humble learners. Maintaining an open attitude to learn from the interviewee works very well with most cultural groups and especially with minorities. It generally reduces status differences between the interviewer and interviewee and makes the cultural minority member feel that he or she has something valuable to share with a representative of another culture. Fear of health professionals (especially Anglo physicians) prevails among many cultural minorities in the United States, often because of their authority and status. Reversing one's role from an expert to a humble learner often takes practice and conscious awareness of one's role. Remaining open to hearing interviewees talk about their cultural myths, religious ideas, folk beliefs, and culturally sensitive areas without expressing demeaning nonverbal or verbal cues to the interviewee is important.

> (8) *Let the interviewee guide the interview, sharing what he or she is comfortable discussing. The interview takes cues from the interviewee, except occasionally to clarify, validate, or direct inquiries about ideas or to open a new domain of inquiry.*

This principle differs from most traditional interviews by health professionals in that the latter tend to *guide the interview* actively. It is an art to get the interviewee to initiate, maintain, and guide the interview. Generally, interviewees from a designated culture know how to tell their ideas *in their cultural style*. If interrupted, the interviewee may not give an accurate account or may lose interest in discussing stories or ideas with the interviewer. The interviewer should try to get the interviewee interested in wanting to tell about his or her world related to the Sunrise Model domains (Figure 5.1). The interviewer takes an active listening and observing role and a passive talking role, and only occasionally clarifies or asks questions, as cultural secrets are seldom shared unless trust prevails.

Interviewees are sensitive to the interviewer's nonverbal behavior and they look for an interviewer to encourage or limit their communication. Verbal statements by the interviewer such as "I would like to hear more about that experience" or "Could you tell me more about your work situation?" are generally open-ended frames and encourage the interviewee to share his or her ideas and experiences.

Throughout the interview, the interviewer should use broad, open-ended areas of inquiry, rather than a series of structured questions that elicit a few words as responses. Some suggested types of interview domains are the following (Spradley, 1979):

> (a) *Broad domains of inquiry:* Initially, one might say, "Would you tell me about yourself, your family, or culture group?" While this may seem to be a very broad domain of inquiry, it encourages the interviewee to talk about any idea within the broad area. Cultural content is not only descriptive, but it contains values, cultural

symbols, historical events, and generally integrated patterns of living. Hence cultural representatives tell things as they know and experience them *from their viewpoints and interpretations*. The interviewer has to get into the interviewee's cultural world as the interviewee describes different events. It is amazing how interviewees with cultural interests favor broad areas to talk about, rather than specific organ, disease, or narrow areas of inquiry that are viewed more as "medical talk." Thus the broad domains permit interviewees to talk about cultural ideas and experiences in their ways rather than in the interviewer's style.

(b) *Clarification and validation inquiries:* To clarify or validate information, the interviewer might say, "I am wondering if you could clarify the idea about the *shaman* helping you get well," or "Could you say why it is a cultural taboo not to eat snake meat during your wife's pregnancy?" These inquiries focus on the area, but allow the interviewee to be more specific. Still another technique is to say something like, "Could you tell me more about your pregnancy taboos?" The "tell me" statement or "it is helpful for me to understand how pregnancy taboos are maintained in your culture" approach allows the interviewee to be the authority on the subject.

(c) *Open-ended inquiries or frames:* Open-ended inquiries or incomplete frames are another way to keep the interview open and to learn about different cultural beliefs or practices from the interviewee. For example, one might say, "You believe that today women in your culture should . . . ?" This open-ended comment permits the interviewee to complete the statement from his or her perspective (the emic view) and to amplify ideas about the topic. Open-ended frames are used to get local definitions and to obtain specific linguistic statements about cultural values, beliefs, and lifeways. In general, these statement help the interviewer get into the world of the interviewee—the emic perspective.

(d) *Inquiries for contrasts of ideas:* In obtaining local or emic data, one could say, "You indicated your child-rearing punishment practices differ considerably from the way your Mexican-American neighbors punish their children. Could you tell me in what ways?" Or, "What are the kinds of punishments you use and how are they different from those of your Mexican-American neighbors?" Or one may ask, "Do you see differences between how a Mexican-American and an Anglo-American mother punishes her child?" These kinds of statements can clarify the interviewee's emic or local view of how the cultural group know and classifies data. Most important, the cultural or native terms are expressed and become known to the interviewer. This approach prevents the interviewer from imposing his or her language, interpretations, or categories upon the interviewee and helps him or her learn about the interviewee's cultural world. Additional questions may be asked if the interviewer is not clear about the differences; but if one listens carefully, one can generally hear the differences or contrasts among ideas expressed.

These are but a few types of inquiry modes for clarification, validation, and contrasts in intercultural interviewing. Additional interview methods can be found in Spradley's book, *The Ethnographic Interview* (1979). There are also other pertinent literature sources covering ethnological and transcultural nursing interview questions or modes of inquiry (Leininger, 1970b, 1978b, 1981b; Pelto, 1970; Spradley, 1970).

(9) *Since the culturological interview primarily seeks to identify behavioral and health lifestyles through identification of cultural values, beliefs, and practices, the interviewer should let the interviewee know this focus and help him or her to feel comfortable with the change from past medical interviews that focused on diseases, illness, and pathological conditions.*

From my experiences, most clients and families tend to believe that "medical" personnel (especially physicians) are interested only in sickness, diseases, symptoms, and treatments. It takes some clear statements to convince the interviewee that nurses (nonmedical) and other health care personnel are interested in other aspects about clients, such as lifestyles, health maintenance, and how individuals and families remain well. If this interest is not known, the interviewee tends to talk about illness and may never talk about cultural values and lifeways. Clients have indeed been socialized to medical norms.

Fortunately, more health professionals and others helping people are beginning to emphasize healthy patterns of living and health maintenance patterns. Thus there is hope that as professional groups shift to healthy patterns of living, clients will know this and feel comfortable talking about their healthy cultural styles of living. In the meantime, the interviewer will need to encourage the client to talk about health that is culturally based. Of course, illness accounts are also culturally based, but the context and way of presenting them are different from the medical modes of inquiry. Ethnographic accounts of health and illness provide refreshing new ways to understand people.

(10) *Clarify the past and current role of the interviewee in order to deter-*
        mine his or her activities, role, and function in the culture.

If one is not aware of the interviewee's role and activities, one may miss his or her key position in the culture. For example, if the interviewee is the mayor of the town, he or she may have many special functions or activities that he or she may want to share with the interviewer, such as resolving political conflicts and health problems with different cultural groups as well as the problems and threats to his or her position. The role of the interviewee should be established early in the interview and should be kept in mind throughout the session, as it provides a valuable frame of reference from which to understand the interviewee.

(11) *During the interview, the interviewer needs to be aware of his or her*
        own verbal and nonverbal responses and mannerisms.

Being sensitive about one's own behavior is critical because as an interviewer one will hear strange ideas one has never heard before. Cultural data about sorcery, witchcraft, or rites of passage for youth may make the interviewer disgusted or uncomfortable. Interviewees are quick to "read" professional reactions to their comments. Interviewers tend to respond nonverbally in many ways, and these responses may be barriers to the ongoing interview. If the interviewee notices a startled reaction to a cultural belief, he or she may suddenly stop sharing ideas, withdraw, or become frightened of potential consequences. When the interviewee notices that the interviewer is uncomfortable or alarmed, he or she can quickly change the discussion. In general, the interviewer must try to main cognizant of his or her behavior and that of the interviewee throughout the interview.

(12) *An the end of an interview, the interviewer should express*
        appreciation to the interviewee for sharing information.

Adherence to this courteous act often makes a difference whether or not the interviewee will return, for it the interviewee has thoughtfully and generously shared his or her ideas, he or she may want to be acknowledged. In addition, common etiquette and courtesy in human relationships often have many beneficial effects.

At any time the interviewee wants to know about the purpose and use of interview data, the interviewer must be willing to clarify this matter. Generally, I have found that interviewees find that telling about their cultural lifeways is important and satisfying; hence return visits have not been difficult to maintain.

Doing a Culturological Assessment and Measuring Outcomes

From the beginning of an intercultural interview, the culturological assessment occurs. The interviewer explores with the interviewee the areas identified on the Sunrise Model and jots down notes based on observations, ideas, and general attitudes identified.

After the interview has been completed, the interviewer (and selected observers) begin to assess particular cultural areas in depth, such as (1) verbal statements; (2) recurrent value themes; (3) patterns of living and dealing with family members and others; (4) interactional patterns of daily living; (5) cultural values, conflicts, and stresses; (6) cultural taboos; (7) social structure features; (8) health-illness system; (9) folk and professional subsystems; and (10) environmental or ecological variables.

Identifying, abstracting, and synthesizing cultural content from the interview takes time and thoughtful deliberation based on data collected. For example, a Navaho interviewee talked about ways to keep healthy by maintaining harmony with the environment. She told about the way people had established taboos so the water and earth would not be polluted and cause illness. This interviewee talked about daily exercises, such as running, to keep her well. She also identified several ideas about the kinship, religions, and political systems that were healthy Navaho lifeways, and others to prevent sickness and witchcraft. Hence themes and patterns of healthy lifeways that are supported by social structure features were identified as guides to nursing therapy. Transcultural nurses operate with themes and patterns of behavior.

In conducting a culturological assessment, it may be difficult to abstract themes or patterns of behavior of the interviewee variables because of the tendency of the interviewer to focus on concrete individual behaviors. In other words, collective patterns of behavior or themes of behavior are difficult to formulate. Identifying themes of behavior abstracted from cultural norms and practices is important. For example, a folk ritual or ceremony is often abstracted from the religious and economic practices of many people. A healing method may be embedded in kinship responsibilities rather than in self-care practices and child rearing may be embedded in political practices.

As one assesses, measures, or determines the weight of the interview, it is important to determine the degree of the interviewee's *acculturation*. A tool I use to determine the degree of acculturation with respect to such cultural variables as language, material goods, family patterns, religious beliefs, kinship patterns, education, technology, and other areas is an interview schedule that has several pages that are used to assess each cultural variable on a five-point traditional versus nontraditional measure or scale. The scale describes a client's acculturation. Each cultural variable is assigned weights. The variables identify areas of variation with respect to cultural variables, themes, and patterns and a profile of therapy goals appropriate to the client. The profile can also stimulate theories, hypotheses, and future research investigations. The cultural variables being assessed are (1) material items (clothing worn, possession symbols), (2) language usage, (3) family cultural patterns, (4) daily life patterns, (5) cultural values expressed, (6) cultural values in action, (7) health beliefs and practices, (8) religious beliefs and values, (9) kinship patterns, (10) political patterns, (11) technological dependency, (12) educational attainment, and (13) other.

At this time, several qualitative and quantitative tools are being explored for culturological assessments or for measurement purposes. Preserving the cultural meaning and other qualitative attributes is an important challenge with these tools. Photographs, autobiographic data, ethnographic themes and other methods of analysis are being used as corroborative modes to obtain an accurate and reliable picture of the individual.

SUMMARY

In this chapter, the rationale for a culturological interview and assessment was presented along with a conceptual framework, practical guidelines, and principles. The culturological interview can be used to determine clients' lifestyles and cultural needs, and for a variety of other purposes. The interview is valuable in determining therapy goals for clients and for teaching, research, and consultation purposes. The culturological interview differs in many ways from most traditional physiological or psychological interviews, and these points of difference were discussed. The potential to build and refine culturological interviews and assessments remains for the future. However, one can expect increasing demands for the use of culturological interviews as health counselors and therapists attempt to provide culture-specific assistance.

Although the focus in this chapter was primarily an individual interview, the reader can use the ideas and the guidelines for families, cultural groups, and community-based interviews. Essentially, the goal has been to increase awareness of the importance of cultural interviews to get into the world of the client as a sound basis to explain, interpret, and predict human behavior and to provide culturally based therapies or assistive services.

APPENDIX:
DEFINITIONS OF BASIC AND KEY TERMS

In this chapter, the following definitions are used:

(1) *Culture* refers to the learned and transmitted knowledge and general lifeways of a designated cultural (or subcultural) group with its particular values, beliefs, and practices (Leininger, 1981b).

(2) *Social structure* refers to the major systems and/or institutionalized units within a society such as the religious, economic, kinship, political, legal, technological, and educational systems that influence and largely determine the cultural lifeways and diverse functioning of a society.

(3) *Intercultural interview* refers to the dynamic process of eliciting information, making observations, and determining actions by an interviewer with respect to culture content provided by an interviewee.

(4) *World view* refers to the perceptions, cognitions, and experiences of individuals (or groups) as they look out upon the world or universe about them.

(5) *Culturological assessment* refers to the process of identifying, abstracting, appraising, and making formulations or judgments about the values, beliefs, and lifeways of an individual (or group) of

a designated culture, with the goal of using this knowledge to provide culturally based health care or related services to people.

(6) *Cultural imposition* refers to the unintended or intended actions of a person caused by placing one's own values, beliefs, and practices upon another person, group, or culture, believing that one's own values or lifeways are the best, most preferred, or superior to others (Leininger, 1981b).

(7) *Cultural preservation* refers to ways of retaining values, beliefs, and practices viewed as advantageous or beneficial to a person or group from a designated culture.

(8) *Cultural accommodation* refers to the creative modes of blending together (or fitting) different cultural values, beliefs, and practices in a different way so an individual or group finds congruence and/or satisfactions with the new or different mode of living.

(9) *Cultural repatterning* refers to the cognitive realignment of different sets of values, beliefs, and practices so a client finds a different way of perceiving and knowing the world.

(10) *Holistic health-illness approach* refers to the conceptual use of social structural and environmental forces as a comprehensive or total picture of a client's health-illness world.

(11) *Folk health subsystem* refers to the roles, functions, and activities of established or traditional local or indigenous carers and curers (healers) prepared by culturally based life experiences, with the goal of helping people maintain health or recover from illness in their natural or familiar environment (Leininger, 1981c).

(12) *Professional health subsystem* refers to the roles, functions, and activities of carers and curers (healers) prepared through formal modes of professional education to provide "modern" or "scientific" professional services to help clients within an institutional frame of reference, that is, hospitals, clinics, and health centers (Leininger, 1981c).

REFERENCES

Cole, M., & Scribner, S. (1973). *Culture and thought: A psychological introduction.* New York: John Wiley.

Draguns, J. G. (1979). Culture and personality. In A. Marsella, R. Tharp, & T. Cifrowski (Eds.), *Perspectives on cross-cultural psychology* (pp. 179-201). New York: Academic.

Leininger, M. (1967). The culture concept and its relevance to nursing. *Journal of Nursing Education, 6,* 27-39.

Leininger, M. (1969). Community psychiatric nursing: Trends, issues and problems. *Perspectives in Psychiatric Care, 1,* 10-20.

Leininger, M. (1970a). Witchcraft practices and nursing therapy. *ANA Clinical Conferences: American Nurses Association Convention in 1969* (pp. 76-80). New York: Appleton-Century-Crofts.

Leininger, M. (1970b). *Nursing and anthropology: Two worlds to blend.* New York: John Wiley.

Leininger, M. (1973) Witchcraft practices and psychocultural therapy with urban United States families. *Human Organization, 32,* 73-83.

Leininger, M. (1976). Cultural interfaces, communication and health implications. In *Proceedings of an Adventure in Transcultural Communication and Health* (pp. 17-21). Honolulu, Hawaii.

Leininger, M. (1978a). *Transcultural nursing: Concepts, theories, and practices.* New York: John Wiley.

Leininger, M. (1978b). Transcultural nursing: A new and scientific subfield of study in nursing. In M. Leininger (Ed.), *Transcultural nursing: Concepts, theories, and practices.* New York: John Wiley.

Leininger, M. (1979). *Transcultural nursing: Proceedings from four national transcultural nursing conferences.* New York: Masson International.

Leininger, M. (Ed.). (1980). *Transcultural nursing: Teaching, research and practice.* Proceedings of the Fifth National Transcultural Nursing Conference, University of Utah. Salt Lake City: Transcultural Nursing Society Press.

Leininger, M. (1981a). Transcultural nursing issues for the 1980's. In J. McCloskey & H. Grace (Eds.), *Current issues in nursing.* Boston: Blackwell Scientific Publications.

Leininger, M. (1981b). *Caring: An essential human need.* Thorofare, Charles B. Slack.

Leininger, M. (1981c, September). Transcultural nursing: Its progress and its future. In National League for Nursing, *Nursing and Health Care.* New York: National League for Nursing.

Leininger, M. (1982). *Transcultural diversity and universality of health and caring: A theory of nursing.* Thorofare, NJ: Charles B. Slack.

Marsella, A. J. (1979). Cross-cultural studies of mental disorders. A. Marsella, R. Tharp, & T. Cebrowski (Eds.), *Perspectives on cross-cultural psychology* (pp. 233-257). New York: Academic.

Marsella, A., & Pedersen, P. (1981). *Cross-cultural counseling and psychotherapy.* Elmsford, NY: Pergamon.

Morley, P. (Ed.). (1981). *Transcultural nursing: Developing, teaching and practicing.* Proceedings of the Sixth National Transcultural Nursing Conference, University of Utah. Salt Lake City: Transcultural Nursing Society Press.

Pelto, P. (1970). *Anthropological research: The structure of inquiry.* New York: Harper & Row.

Spradley, B. W. (1982). *Readings in community health nursing* (2nd ed.). Boston: Little, Brown.

Spradley, J. (1970). *You owe yourself a drunk: An ethnography of urban nomads.* Boston: Little, Brown.

Spradley, J. (1979). *The ethnographic interview.* New York: Holt, Rinehart & Winston.

6

DELIVERING MENTAL HEALTH SERVICES ACROSS CULTURES

HARRIET P. LEFLEY

INTRODUCTION

Expansion of mental health service delivery systems at local, national, and international levels has raised a broad spectrum of issues that relate, essentially, to the reliability and validity of existing models of care. Within Western nations we are seeing a testing of new therapeutic approaches and innovative service models, largely as a result of community mental health ideology and the extension of services to low-income, multiethnic, and newly acculturating populations. There are multiple issues relating to service delivery, but perhaps the most salient are the following: (a) integration of traditional psychiatric concepts of mental health services with the more global community mental health approaches—in both technologically advanced and developing nations; (b) cross-national and cross-cultural relevance and potential for implementation of service models developed in Western countries; (c) appropriate attitudes toward and utilization of already existing healing systems; (d) development of culturally sensitive service delivery models for immigrant or transplanted populations at varying levels of acculturation; and (e) effects of cross-cultural research findings on current levels of knowledge and future development plans.

The pattern of modern mental health care has largely been dominated by two historical events. One, the pharmacologic revolu-

AUTHOR'S NOTE: The author would like to thank Mrs. Carmen B. Rivera for her invaluable bibliographic and typing assistance. Special acknowledgment is due Dr. Mercedes Sandoval for her contributions to the discussion of folk healing.

tion, has been instrumental in depopulating the mental hospitals of most Western countries. This has been accompanied by a philosopical revolution that (a) disputed the validity of the concept of mental illness on epistemological grounds (Szasz, 1974); (b) postulated countertherapeutic effects due to institutionalization, a clear violation of the Hippocratic oath to do no harm (Goffman, 1962); and (c) developed a rationale for a spectrum of services that would treat all levels of mental disorder, at the primary, secondary, and teritary levels of prevention, within the community setting (Caplan, 1964).

In the United States, these philosophic currents were moved forward rapidly by the passage of the Community Mental Health Centers Act of 1963, which proposed to offer easily accessible, quality mental health care in a nationwide network of community facilities. With a mandate to deliver inpatient, outpatient, day treatment, and crisis emergency care, as well as consultation and education, the centers were later required to add substance-abuse treatment, court screening, specialized services for children and the elderly, and aftercare and transitional housing for previously hospitalized patients. Thus the package of mandated services was, it seemed, comprehensive enough to encompass all contingencies.

This comprehensive approach was developmentally related to the emergence in the late 1960s of what Schulberg (1977) has termed a "community mental health ideology." Its core concepts included responsibility for the care of all potentially disabled members of a community, primary prevention, social treatment goals, continuity of care, and total community involvement. The focus was similar to Mehryar and Khajavi's (1974, p. 45) proposal of a community mental health model for developing countries:

> An open systems conceptualization of the whole process of the organization and delivery of mental health services [that] will help bring about an integration of mental health services within the wider framework of human services agencies, e.g., public health, general and adult education, family planning, and community development.

The key features are an emphasis on primary prevention, paraprofessional training, consultation and education, and development of community alternatives to hospitalization. Some of the primary prevention features suggested in the model are being applied today, independently, in developing countries. An example is a pilot mental health project in Honduras, devised by Dr. Alfredo Padilla, Chief of Mental Health in the Ministry of Public Health and Social Assistance, in which residents of a poor community were organized, in a multilevel consciousness-raising process, into goal-directed groups for mutual self-help and resolution of common social and environmental problems (Eisenberg, 1980).

 In the United States, there is an increasing trend toward affiliation agreements between community mental health centers (CMHCs) and neighborhood health centers. These affiliations are typically based on two levels of integration: specific linkage services and conjoint services. In some CMHCs, such as the New Horizons center described in this chapter, the linkage is limited to a special mental health services unit within a primary health care clinic, while the freestanding CMHC continues to provide mental health services as a specialized entity. In a comprehensive overview of the linkage model, Borus et al. (1980) describe a network of 850 community health centers in operation throughout the United States, which, unlike freestanding mental health delivery sites, offer a "one-stop" setting for conjoint health and mental health care. In addition to offering a holistic approach and a comprehensive service package, the integrated model avoids the stigmatization of mental health patients as a unique consumer category, thus enhancing acceptability of services.

 A parallel, but more comprehensive, trend is exemplified in the new Italian system in which Maxwell Jones's therapeutic community concept has been translated into a complete spectrum of community mental health care. According to psychiatrists Paolo Tranchino of the Psychiatric Public Services of Florence and Agostino Pirella, Superintendent of Psychiatric Services in Turin, the merger of biological, psychological, and sociological disciplines has resulted in a broad-based community care system that ranges from locating housing for patients in the community to convincing the public to accept them (ADAMHA, 1981). National reform legislation passed in 1978 and implemented in 1980 imposed a total ban on the building of new psychiatric hospitals, with most patients entering the psychiatric wards of general hospitals in the event of an acute psychotic episode. Largely the result of a lifetime of work by pioneering psychiatrist Franco Basaglia, the Italian emphasis on deinstitutionalization, decentralization, and total community care closely parallels current ideological trends in the United States (Miller, Mazade, Muller, & Andrulis, 1978), England (Wing, 1980), France (Gittelman, Dubuis, & Gillet, 1973), and the Scandinavian countries (Kringlen, 1981).

Problems with the
Community Mental Health Model

   Although the open systems approach is proving increasingly attractive, a number of theoretical and empirical problems have arisen in implementing the comprehensive service model in the United States. Some of the more critical issues include (a) the conceptual scope of mental health services, (b) service priorities, (c) equitable allocation of professional and paraprofessional resources, (d) concepts of prevention and the prevention/treatment cost-benefit ratio, and (e) degree and nature of community participation.
   The first issue is, of course, the most basic. In the years when mental health professionals shuttled between hospital and private practice, limiting their services to clear diagnostic categories, there was little attention to the vast behavioral problem area engendered by social disruption. Today, with the development of some of the types of programs described in this chapter, questions arise as to whether, for example, community organization is a legitimate mental health function; whether provision of social outlets for lonely but functional elderly (Ross, 1975) is a valid service priority; whether centers have neglected the severely mentally ill in order to serve the "merely unhappy" (Lamb, 1977); and whether mental health planning without adequate political and economic support can have any impact on social decompensation.
   Since the community mental health model vastly expands the number of potential service recipients, a major issue relates to priorities and allocation of resources to treatment of the severely mentally ill. As hospitalized patients, their legitimacy as a priority target group was unquestioned. In the community, however, it is apparent that many community mental health centers have neglected the needs of the chronic patient (Hogarty, 1971; Kirk & Therrien, 1975). Dealing with chronic patients is related to staff burnout and low job satisfaction (Pines & Maslach, 1978), and is perceived as low yield for a heavy investment of time and effort (Lamb, 1977). It is ironic, for example, that while hospital care and partial hospitalization were mandated services in the 1963 CMHC legislation, aftercare, added a decade later, could almost be interpreted as an afterthought (see Glasscote, 1975). In a 25-year follow-up of Hollingshead and Redlich's (1958) study on social class and mental illness, Mollica and Redlich (1980) reported on the current treatment

settings for patient groups that in 1950 either were totally excluded from psychiatric care or were using the state hospital exclusively. They found that despite an enormous proliferation in range and number of available psychiatric services, in 1975 such patients were still receiving their inpatient care at the state hospital or in outpatient units characterized by low-intervention treatment and staffed by semiprofessional or nonprofessional clinicians. This highlights the question of equity for such "low-status" patients within the mental health delivery system.

The ratio of preventive to direct treatment services is an especially critical issue in low-income multiproblem areas where groups at high risk for decompensation may dwell side by side with deinstitutionalized former mental patients (Levy & Rowitz, 1973) who need ongoing outpatient care. Equitable investment of resources thus hinges on the question of whether our present level of technology permits us to determine whether a psychopathology can actually be prevented. While there is a literature indicating relative reduction in the expected frequencies of new cases as a result of interventions (Munoz, 1976), these studies typically refer to very moderate forms of behavioral disorder and do not involve substantive long-range findings. Whether and how psychosis can be prevented remains the domain of multicultural, longitudinal research. Thus the allocation of funds to preventive efforts (primarily consultation and education) versus direct treatment to an identified patient population is constantly being debated, without any firm basis for evaluation.

Allocation of professional and paraprofessional resources is a related issue. In the community mental health centers, scarce psychiatrists spend most of their time on medication evaluation, while psychotherapy is left to other disciplines and, often, to paraprofessionals. Despite the multiple problems outlined with respect to psychotherapy with multiethnic populations, minority groups often complain that their care is left to indigenous paraprofessionals, an inference that Mollica and Redlich's (1980) data tend to confirm. This factor is viewed as further evidence of institutional racism (see Gaviria & Stern, 1980).

A further critical issue is the planning and decision-making function. In the United States, community mental health centers are directed by governing boards mandated by law to represent the catchment area demographically in terms of age, sex, and ethnicity. Since members are citizen rather than consumer representatives, many board laypersons must go through a long period of orientation and education in mental health issues before they are knowledgeable enough to be useful. The relationship between professional staff and their lay employers and the potential for political manipulation and power struggles are factors affecting the service delivery system.

At the social planning level, issues are further compounded by conflicting priorities of different interest groups. For example, the consistent underutilization of mental health services by Hispanics in the United States has generated intense interest in rendering services more culturally appropriate and acceptable for this group. Gaviria and Stern (1980) describe three constituencies active in planning services for Hispanics, with each approaching the issue from a different perspective: Government funding agencies stress geographic proximity; social scientists highlight the need to recognize indigenous folk belief systems and practitioners; and Hispanic community activists see the key to cultural relevance in provision of bicultural, bilingual staff. These three constituencies involved in planning and delivering mental health services have frequently clashed, and Gaviria and Stern report that actual changes in service delivery have been difficult to implement.

Cross-Cultural Research
and Service Utilization in the United States

The repeated stricture against transplanting the traditional psychiatric model to developing countries receives confirmation from the experiences of different ethnic groups in the West. Here, there are numerous cultural barriers to utilization of the mental health delivery system. Some of these barriers are institutional, while others are a function of cultural definitions of appropriate and inappropriate behavior, belief systems, attitudes, and values.

In the United States, a history of institutional racism has effectively barred minority group members from higher education and professional training. As a result, despite affirmative action policies and growing availability of mental health services to low-income, multiethnic clients, the typical service provider remains white, middle class, and non-Hispanic. The experiential and cognitive distance between such service providers and the average catchment area client has generated a wide range of difficulties. These include linguistic barriers in evaluating psychopathology (Marcos & Alpert,

1976); underrecording or misinterpretation of symptoms (De Hoyos & De Hoyos, 1965); arbitrary criteria for emergency commitment (Peszke & Winthrob, 1974); serious diagnostic errors (Simon et al., 1973); failure to understand differential response patterns on screening instruments (Gynther, 1972); basic communication difficulties and bias in interviewing (Carkhuff & Pierce, 1967); misinterpretation of psychodynamics (Thomas & Sillen, 1972); advice that is counter to cultural mores (Lombillo & Geraghty, 1973); failure to differentiate between adaptive and maladaptive behavior (Abad, Ramos, & Boyce, 1974); and limitations in client self-disclosure (Acosta & Sheehan, 1978).

The net result has been differential treatment and outcome, together with a demonstration of massive avoidance behavior on the part of mental health professionals. Research indicates that nonwhite, non-Anglo patients are more likely to receive arbitrary diagnoses based on limited or ambiguous recording of symptomatology, are less often accepted for psychotherapy, are more often assigned to inexperienced therapists, are seen for shorter periods of time, and are more likely to receive either supportive or custodial care, or drugs alone (see Lefley, 1974, for overview).

The cultural barriers are, of course, bilateral. If mental health professionals tend to avoid patients from contrast cultures, the latter are even more likely to avoid the orthodox mental health establishment. Major barriers to utilization in the developing countries are similar to those found in multicultural enclaves in the United States: the social stigma of modern psychiatry, particularly fear of hospitalization; a lack of confidence in modern psychiatry; the strength of belief systems; the availability of alternate healers; and the relationships between alternate healers and the Western system (see Higginbotham, 1979). In the United States, underutilization is particularly pronounced among minorities. In a study of nearly 14,000 patients in 17 community mental health centers in the Northwest over a three-year period, Sue (1977) found that about half of all ethnic minority clients (Black, Asian-American, Chicano, and Native American) failed to return after one session. Similar findings were reported by Andrulis (1977).

Concurrent with the emergent findings on cultural service barriers to lower socioeconomic ethnic patients has been the parallel body of data suggesting that it is precisely such groups, overrepresented among the poor, who might need mental health services the most. By now the data seem clear that the lowest socioeconomic groups have the highest rates of severe psychiatric disorder (Dohrenwend et al., 1980), and that in the United States hospitalization for mental illness appears to increase during economic recessions and decrease during economic upturns (Brenner, 1973). Thus, putting aside etiological questions, there seems to be impressive correlational evidence that social-environmental stressors may exacerbate preexisting conditions, trigger mental health crises among the vulnerable and their families, and/or create a negative ambience affecting child-rearing and family transactions.

These parallel bodies of research findings have influenced the development of multilevel models of service delivery to lower-income multicultural communities in the United States, particularly in large urban centers with immigrant populations. One of these models, incorporating systems modification and culturally sensitive therapeutic modalities, will be described more fully in the section on service delivery models.

CULTURAL VALUES AND COMMUNITY CARE FOR THE MENTALLY ILL

In every country, the mental health delivery system must deal with a chronic or potentially chronic population. At this point in history, the pharmacologic revolution has generated a worldwide capability for reducing hospital populations and resettling the mentally ill in the community. Hailed as a civil libertarian and fiscal triumph, this permits the provision of a lower-cost "least restrictive setting" for people who are, after all, noncriminal but require sheltered care. The presumed bankruptcy of this effort in the United States has been discussed at great length, both in the popular press and in the scientific literature (Bachrach, 1978; Committee on Psychiatry and the Community, 1978), and in television programs. Similar problems have been reported in England (Korer, Freeman, & Cheadle, 1978). In brief, deinstitutionalization has taken place without commensurate community resources, and the creation of "mental health ghettos" in the depressed inner city and isolated outlying areas has frequently re-created an institutional ambience while stripping patients of hospital supports.

In the United States, reports on the progress of deinstitutionalization indicate that long-term patients have been shortchanged by the very movement that was designed to ease their plight. Bachrach (1978) suggests a general consensus that the planning for community mental health centers was geared toward persons who could for the most part look out for themselves—a fact embodied in the failure of the 1963 legislation to require follow-up care or transitional housing. The President's Commission on Mental Health (1978) has reported that often the only community-based treatment offered to chronic patients is medication.

A wide range of sheltered-care models have evolved over the years (Budson, 1979), with a concomitant growth of the psychosocial rehabilitation movement. However, evaluative studies have indicated highly inconclusive findings on the success of community placement (Carpenter, 1978). As Bachrach (1978) points out, we have not yet attained sufficient historical perspective to determine the success or failure of this massive change in services for the severely disabled.

Currently in the United States a counterpart population of young adult chronic patients (aged 18-35) is joining the deinstitutionalized group as candidates for services in the community. As a result of strict legal requirements for involuntary commitment, and the current tendencies of hospitals to reject or limit the stay of all but the most floridly psychotic, many of these young adults have gone numerous times through the "revolving door" of the emergency room or crisis intervention unit without actually having been institutionalized. Persistently dysfunctional, they may overuse outpatient facilities without problem resolution for many years, while continuing to live with their families as dependent children (Pepper, Kirshner, & Ryglewicz, 1981). A similar situation obtains in the Federal Republic of Germany, where Haase (1981) maintains that since the introduction of phenothiazines in the 1950s only one out of every two persons with schizophrenia ever undergoes inpatient treatment in a psychiatric hospital. These ex-hospitalized and never-hospitalized individuals thus constitute a patient pool requiring ongoing comprehensive care in the community.

Community Support:
Lessons from Cross-Cultural Research

In our multifaceted approach to aftercare services, most Western commentators have not yet made the conceptual leap from the medical model (professional ministrations) to creation of a viable community lifestyle for the mentally ill. There is still a conceptual separation between aftercare, which is limited to medication and continuing psychotherapy, and "case management," which applies to services that provide housing, income, and vocational and social rehabilitation (Talbott, 1981).

While there is an increasing emphasis on residential programs (Lamb et al., 1976; Pepper et al., 1981) and on skill building rather than therapy as a major component of psychosocial rehabilitation (Anthony, 1977), a major barrier stems not from professional ethnocentrism but from a world view actively in conflict with the needs of the chronically ill. The single overarching principle informing our aftercare policy in the United States today derives from what Hsu (1972) has called the "American core value," that is, fear of dependency and emphasis on self-reliance. Throughout the literature on psychosocial rehabilitation, the phrase "return the patient to independent living" appears over and over again. For the many chronic patients who never functioned independently, and for those whose skills have been eroded by illness, idleness, or institutionalization, this objective may be not only unrealistic but countertherapeutic. Emphasis on self-reliance carries over into psychotherapy, where a major thrust has been to loosen dependency ties on significant others. When patients require rehospitalization, the tendency is to truncate treatment on theoretical as well as financial grounds—since too long a stay may again incur dependency. Day treatment programs and psychosocial rehabilitation centers traditionally have had high-expectancy objectives. The terms for services imply linguistically the expectation of linear progress: "transitional," "halfway," and "step-level."

The frequent reports of anxiety and unwillingness to leave on the part of the residents in transitional community care (for example, see Wing, 1975), suggest that in many cases this orientation asks far too much of patients, and may exacerbate precisely those feelings that are central to their illness—anxiety and apartness. It also imposes, as a matter of policy, a built-in impermanence in the lives of people who may require long-term stability in order to remain intact.

The subject of dependency is rarely noted, except as a pathological sign, in the research literature of the West. In the clinical literature, there has been a marked failure to differentiate between neurotic dependency as an intrapsychic phenomenon and interpersonal dependency as a socially adaptive mechanism—a failure with ramifications for the items used in screening instruments and for assessments of family dynamics. As a case in point, Guthrie's (1966) cross-cultural studies of the factorial structure of maternal child-rearing attitudes have indicated, for example, that "dependency in North America refers to a fear of self-assertion and a longing for support, while in the Philippines it may refer to strong family integration. Guthrie found that fostering dependency in the Philippines was related to family support and responsibility, while in the United States it was related to maternal control and authority. Using the same instrument, I also found significant differences in the positive/negative valence of dependency in two American Indian tribes at different levels of social integration (Lefley, 1976). Other cross-cultural research comparing data from the Bahamas, Thailand, and the Philippines (Lefley, 1972, 1976) has suggested that Western sanctions against expressing dependency needs in childhood may produce strong needs for affiliation in adulthood.

The major work of dependency, of course, has been that of Doi (1969, 1973). Unlike Freud, who related dependency to libidinal satisfaction, Doi has postulated that dependency is the primordial drive of all humankind. The manner in which a society resolves this drive affects the world view, transactions, productivity, and mental health of its members. The Japanese concept of amae appears to express a cultural norm of interdependence and selective indulgence of weaknesses, in contrast to the Western ideal of self-reliance and nonindulgence. Similarly, Phillips's (1965) description of the bilateral nature of dependency in the relationship between social inferiors and superiors in Thailand suggests a societally sanctioned reciprocity that leaves everyone with self-respect.

These issues are highly germane to the lonely, isolated, dysfunctional lives of many former patients who have been "returned to independent living" in the urban communities of the West. Apart from their symptoms, ex-patients are typically immobilized by two critical variables: (a) lack of a human support system and (b) feelings of worthlessness and low self-esteem. A societal value structure that idealizes individualism, fails to support the notion of group interdependence, and withholds respect from the dysfunctional does much to reinforce the toxic labeling process that Waxler (1974, 1979) related to chronicity.

Today, there is some indication of a movement away from the "transitional," or "halfway," concept in England (Soni, Soni, & Freeman, 1978) toward the recognition that housing for the disabled must be long term or even permanent. In Norway and Sweden a certain percentage of new housing is set aside for ex-patients, with plans proposed in France and Denmark (Gittelman, 1978).

In the ARO village system developed by Lambo (1966) in Nigeria and now extended to Senegal (Collomb, 1978), patients live with a relative in a traditional village close to the mental hospital or clinic. Treatment is organically related to village life, incorporating both traditional and Western therapies (psychotropic medication and group therapy). Lambo's (1978) emphasis on the community's role in healing as an integral part of society and religion and the therapeutic aspects of "community ethos" in China (Sidel & Sidel, 1972) contradict what is presumed to be the key element of successful case outcome in the West, that is, the personal relationship between patient and therapist.

Several projects have emerged in the United States that attempt to involve the ex-patient in a living community system. Merging group support with the American core value is the Fairweather Lodge system, now evaluating 25 years of implementation (Fairweather, 1980). This is a work-residence model that has moved hundreds of patients out of the hospital into small peer-controlled living units with the aim of developing a self-sustaining economic base.

The Foster Community Project in Missouri (Fields, 1974), designed as a model for integrating chronic psychiatric patients into small towns, was developed partially in the Geel tradition, with the aim of developing foster colonies that would benefit economically and psychologically through offering homes to chronic psychiatric patients. Several foster communities have been successfully developed in rural areas. Unfortunately, such aftercare projects are few and far between. Even in the Community Support Program of the National Institute of Mental Health, aftercare treatment has rarely made provision for human support networks (as opposed to case management) as part of the formal treatment plan, despite a renewal of interest in this topic for schizophrenic patients (Schizophrenia Bulletin, 1981).

Yet there is a strong suggestion in the cross-cultural literature of the efficacy of such networks in preventing decompensation both within the United States (Garrison, 1978) and cross-nationally (Waxler, 1979; Westermeyer & Pattison, 1981). In particular, the findings of the International Pilot Study of Schizophrenia (IPSS) of a more benign outcome and better prognosis for insidious-onset schizophrenics in developing countries (Sartorius, Jablensky, & Shapiro,

1978) is viewed as presumptive evidence that supportive kinship networks, together with the less stressful life of uncomplicated societies, provide a protective environment that impedes development of illness and aids in recovery (Mosher & Keith, 1981). In the view of Mosher and Keith (1981), the low stress-high support hypothesis is further confirmed by the life stress (Brown, Birley, & Wing, 1972) and expressed emotion (Vaughn & Leff, 1976) studies from the United Kingdom. These findings are increasingly being utilized in clinical training of mental health professionals. This cross-cultural research, also, lends considerable support to the psychosocial rehabilitation service model that is rapidly supplanting or augmenting traditional psychiatric aftercare treatment.

The Family in the Service Network

Parallel to the IPSS findings is the emergent realization that community care has generated an empirical need for families' participation in the service network, both as primary caregiver, where this is feasible, and as basic support system for the patient. In the cross-cultural literature on patient care there are indications that in nonindustrial societies, where families typically accompany the patient and often wait out the hospitalization period in close proximity to the clinic, the family is often seen as an asset (Jegende, 1981) or may even be engaged in a therapeutic role (Lambo, 1966).

This is in sharp contrast to the negative view of many Western mental health professionals who have implicated families as etiologic agents. By rejecting family members and ignoring their requests for information and help, professionals have often alienated the very support systems that patients seem to need for benevolent outcome (Goldstein, 1981). A historical conjunction of events seems to be changing such attitudes. With deinstitutionalization, over 65 percent of psychiatric inpatients in the United States return to live with their families (Goldman, 1982). Concurrently, several lines of research tend to suggest that negative family role, when perceived, may be correlative or reactive rather than causal. One stems from findings in biological/genetic psychiatry that point to diathesis, another from research on family burden in the care of mentally ill persons that indicates profound and periodically intolerable stress (Arey &

Wahrheit, 1980; Hatfield, 1978; Wing, 1975). At the same time, the expressed emotion (EE) studies, which demonstrate a relationship between critical overinvolvement and relapse, also reveal a large number of low-EE families who provide benign support for schizophrenic members. Emergent cross-cultural findings even suggest that high EE may be quite atypical in traditional cultures (Day, 1982; Karno, 1982). A *zeitgeist* is emerging that makes it propitious for professionals to make alliances with the primary caregivers.

In recent years there has been an attempt to counteract the effects of the concept of the schizophrenogenic patient, a concept that has filtered down through the popular media and that tends to alienate already frustrated and overstressed family systems. Because of the literature on communication deviance, clinicians still focus on family dynamics and disturbed communication when involving relatives in treatment. Nevertheless, there is increasing questioning of (a) the family therapy orientation that seeks to label all members as patients (Lamb & Oliphant, 1978) and (b) failure of professionals to recognize family pain and burden as a legitimate stressor and independent high-risk concern (Arey & Wahrheit, 1980; Goldman, 1982; Hatfield, 1978; Wing, 1975).

In this connection, two new currents in the service delivery system should be noted. First, there is increasing acceptance by mental health professionals of intervention strategies such as (a) organizing multiple-family support groups and (b) providing psychoeducational interventions to teach families about schizophrenia or manic-depressive illness and how to manage patients' behavior, rather than traditional family therapy (Beels & McFarlane, 1982). Second, national organizations of families of chronic mental patients have developed in several countries—the National Schizophrenia Foundation in England (Wing, 1975) and, currently, the National Alliance for the Mentally Ill in the United States. These organizations have added mutual self-help groups to the service armamentarium. Also, through ongoing education and publicity, working with psychosocial rehabilitation programs, and advocating for needed legislation, these groups facilitate a higher level of community care for chronic patients.

CROSS-CULTURAL RESEARCH AND
SERVICE DELIVERY MODELS

We have previously indicated the emergent impact of the IPSS findings on conceptual models of aftercare, particularly in the development of supportive networks for schizophrenic patients. Within the United States, research on Kluckhohn and Strodtbeck's (1961) value orientations has affected cross-cultural service delivery models in the Boston area among Italian, Greek, Puerto Rican, and other families (Papajohn & Spiegel, 1975) and on cultural training given mental health professionals in the Brandeis University Ethnicity and Mental Health Project (Spiegel, 1981). Similarly, a study of cross-cultural value orientations among Cuban, Haitian, Puerto Rican, Bahamian, and Southern Black families in the University of Miami's Health Ecology Project (Egeland, 1978), described below, has led to interventions based on such temporal and relational variables as present-time orientation, greater directiveness, therapist self-disclosure, and the like (Lefley & Bestman, 1982). Value orientations have also been used in the work of the Spanish Family Guidance Center with Hispanic-American youths (Szapocznik, Scopetta, & King, 1978).

The Spanish-Speaking Mental Health Research Center at the University of California has been instrumental in developing pluralistic counseling approaches with Hispanics, particularly Mexican-Americans (Miranda, 1976; Padilla, 1981). Delgado and Scott (1979) and Ruiz (1977) have contributed greatly to our knowledge of therapy with Puerto Ricans. Sandoval (1977, 1979), at the University of Miami's New Horizons CMHC, has developed a number of innovative approaches integrating folk beliefs with standard therapeutic modalities among Cubans, Puerto Ricans, and other Hispanics. The Spanish Family Guidance Center at the University of Miami has utilized a number of different therapeutic approaches for Miami Cubans. The most recent is the development of bicultural effectiveness training (BET) as a therapeutic modality. This is an empirically derived approach based on findings of a biculturalism and cultural involvement scale (Szapocznik, Kurtines,

& Fernandez, 1980). Validated on Cuban Hispanics, the scale demonstrated lower levels of adjustment at both ends of the continuum, that is, among underacculturated and overacculturated youth. BET incorporates ethnic values clarification and is specifically geared toward enhancing communication and negotiation skills necessary for living in both Hispanic and North American cultural worlds.

Several interest service delivery models evolved from the work of Woodbury (1969), a psychiatrist who has been involved in mental health planning in the Caribbean for many years. The models were originally developed by Woodbury and his wife, a social worker, in France, and were subsequently utilized in the Virgin Islands and in Puerto Rico. These involved a system of community-centered psychiatric interventions with the use of mobile emergency units including home visiting teams and indigenous homemakers (see Ruiz, Vazquez, & Vazquez, 1973, for the use of mobile units among multicultural populations in New York). Two therapeutic modalities emerging from these *in situ* team interventions were (a) the "continuous group" and (b) the "multiple-family group." The continuous group is actually a family walk-in clinic offering patients and their families crisis intervention and group therapy "on demand." The multiple-family group is a variant of family-group psychotherapy, in which families with problems become therapists for other families with problems, rather like the extension of self-help groups with clinical backup. "All members learn rather quickly our basic techniques of psychotherapy and are expected . . . to participate in the resolution of one another's conflicts. . . . They are encouraged to assist one another in their neighborhood without our mediation. . . . Family treats family" (Woodbury, 1969, p. 70).

A Systems Approach:
The University of Miami-New Horizons Model

In this section, I will describe a systems approach to culturally appropriate services that has incorporated many of the features separately outlined by Higginbotham (1976, 1979) for planning a culture-specific mental health service delivery system. This process was based on a conceptual model that similarly began with a search for emic definitions (Weidman, 1975) and has developed empirically on a trial-and-error basis in an attempt to be responsive to community needs.

The University of Miami-Jackson Memorial Medical Center Community Mental Health Center, now the New Horizons CMHC, evolved from a three-year research effort entitled the Health Ecology Project (Weidman, 1978). Codirected by Dr. Hazel Weidman, a social anthropologist, and Dr. James Sussex, psychiatry chairman, the project investigated health beliefs, systems, and behavior among five major ethnic groups in Miami: Bahamians, Cubans, Haitians, Puerto Ricans, and U.S. Southern Blacks. Preliminary findings suggested culturally patterned differences in the clustering of symptoms, culture-bound syndromes with a large psychogenic overlay, unrecognized by orthodox medical or mental health professions (Lefley, 1979a; Weidman, 1979), and the wide use of altenative healing modalities. Field interviews and daily health calendars indicated a high degree of emotional stress for which clinical mental health treatment was neither solicited nor countemplated. In sum, the findings strongly suggested that a community mental health center established along traditional psychiatric lines would be neither maximally effective nor optimally utilized.

The CMHC model, initiated in 1974, began with a dual mandate: (a) to provide culturally sensitive services to its multiethnic catchment area, and (b) to assure that the impoverished communities received their fair share of adaptive resources. The program began with the innovative deployment of five teams of mental health workers, one for each of the ethnic groups previously mentioned. Extensive mapping of the area indicated that the balance of the population most in need of services was elderly, primarily Anglo and U.S. Black. For these target groups two geriatric teams were then developed. Each team is composed of staff, both professional and paraprofessional, who for the most part are of the same cultural extraction as the populations they serve.

Teams, composed of neighborhood workers, mental health technicians, and professional clinicians, are directed by professional social scientists. These team directors are called "culture brokers"— a professional role in the health care delivery system first developed by Weidman (1973), involving a bridging, teaching, and training function at the interface of the hospital and community, and within the two systems. Culture brokers are members of the Department of Psychiatry and have combined academic, applied social scientists, and service provider roles. The teams maintain a network of clinics in the seven communities they serve, with regular and rotating clinical staff including part-time psychiatrists, psychologists, clinical social workers, and nurses.

During its eight years, the CMHC has offered a wide range of decentralized preventive, therapeutic, and supportive outpatient and social/rehabilitative services in the community. Team functions, in addition to traditional chemotherapy and psychotherapy, have included neighborhood outreach programs and massive community entry efforts, beginning with needs assessment to determine culturally defined mental health problems. These have been followed by case finding and resource linkages; community-based consultation and education; direct services in homes, churches, board and care homes, and the like; development of supportive networks for social isolates; programmatic research, including ethnographic and demographic profiles; and community organization and development. In this connection, teams have acted as initiators and coordinators of various projects to bring new resources into their communities or strengthen existing ones; conducted action research to provide supportive data for needed social programs, such as day-care centers, hot lunches for the elderly, and the like; linked consumer groups with appropriate service agencies; and helped residents learn how to utilize resources to ameliorate environmental problems.

The teams work with the patient in an ecological context, within the concentricity of family, neighborhood support system, and community resource networks. They have also be particularly active in the catalyst role of mobilizing consumers to achieve mastery over their lives through community organization. (The entire August 1975 issue of *Psychiatric Annals* was devoted to a description of this program. See especially Lefley, 1975b; Sandoval & Tozo, 1975; Weidman, 1975, for the initial model; see Lefley, 1979b; Lefley & Bestman, 1982, for its history and current status.)

Originally linked with a large country hospital, the culture broker's role has always involved consultation and cultural interpretation. In teaching mental health and medical staff about a particular culture, the culture broker focused not only on those beliefs and practices that may impinge on effective mental health care delivery, but also on adaptive strategies, strengths, and structural supportive elements that may be applied to the preventive model. The role may involve explaining the "rooted" or "hexed" patient to a crisis emergency room nurse unable to diagnose the observed symptoms within the traditional noseology. It may involve teaching psychiatric residents how to differentiate between legitimate paranoid ideation—that is, ideas that are considered bizarre in the culture—from ideation that would be considered in the "normal" range within its conceptual framework. It might involve informing an intake worker that certain requests may be perfectly acceptable to a white, middle-class patient—such as, asking a wife to bring her husband in for counseling—but would generally be unacceptable in certain Hispanic cultures, in which a respected older family member might be a more appropriate intermediary (see Lombillo & Geraghty, 1973). Conversely, the culture broker may facilitate understanding and utilization of services by the ethnic patients within the context of his or her belief systems.

Development of culturally appropriate treatment is an ongoing empirical process, beginning with therapists who can communicate both linguistically and culturally with their clients. The range of modalities has included the following: (a) a network of culturally homogeneous "miniclinics" in seven different communities, many of which function also as "drop-in" neighborhood centers, permitting a patient-community mix; (b) home visits and family consultation in nonthreatening social settings; (c) group therapy within a social-recreational context, such as a painting or macrame class; (d) involvement of extended family in therapy; (e) group meditation and body awareness; (f) merger of traditional and modern healing techniques; (g) consultation and referral to folk healers as needed. Evaluation data have indicated that this approach seems to work, with high client satisfaction, good therapeutic outcome, and significantly lower "no-show" and dropout rates than would be expected based on comparative and baseline data (Lefley & Bestman, 1982).

FOLK HEALING:
LEVELS OF INTEGRATION

Contemporary accounts of mental health systems strongly suggest that even today, in both the developing and technologically advanced countries, mental disorder is frequently perceived in terms of supernatural causation or spirit possession (Delgado, 1979; Erinosho, 1979; Higginbotham, 1979; Holdstock, 1979; Kapur, 1979; Sandoval, 1979; Snyder, 1981).

In developing countries, modern psychiatry is largely associated with chemotherapy, ECT, and hospital confinement. Modern trained practitioners are numerically fewer and geographically localized, and offer an arcane etiology and technology that is culturally incomprehensible to many service recipients. Above all, the stigma of hospitalization carries a greater labeling potential than the transient crisis of spirit possession. Thus in most countries modern practitioners compete with a ubiquitous mass of folk healers for the care of the mentally ill.

In Nigeria, Uyanga (1979) notes that spiritual healing churches have proliferated despite tremendous improvements in hospitals and health care delivery. Tandem usage of folk healers and modern practitioners offers no conflict (Delgado, 1979; Koss, 1980; Weidman, 1978). Most writers on the subject strongly advocate consultation with native healers, for example, Holdstock (1979; South Africa) Kapur (1979; rural India), Koss (1980; Puerto Rico), and many others. Draguns (1981, p. 5) has noted that in the current World Health Organization project to organize community-based mental health services in four developing countries, the "blending in of native psychotherapy is an important component."

Interestingly, but not unpredictably, there seems to be a growing interest in utilizing the services of folk healers among Western mental health professionals, while reluctance is found among those whose training in modern methods is relatively recent. Several departments of psychiatry and other official health providers in highly industrialized urban centers in the United States have encouraged or established linkages with folk healers (Delgado, 1979; Garrison, 1977; Koss, 1980; Ruiz & Langrod, 1976; Lefley & Bestman, 1982; Rodriguez & Hernandex, 1979; Sandoval, 1979; Walton & Curet, 1979; Weidman, 1978, 1979).

Higginbotham (1979, p. 533), however, found a contrasting set of responses when querying mental health professionals in Taiwan, the Philippines, and Thailand. He reports:

> Although there was solid agreement that staff should know the folk healing practices for mental disorder, in no instance was native folk healer participation sought in case management. Most, in fact, eschew folk doctor involvement. They view it as a waste of finances, a delay from proper care, or even harmful. Staff will ask that families stop taking their ailing members to indigenous practitioners while under psychiatric care. When staff feel that such visits interfere with their own therapeutics, they insist on discontinuation of healer contact.

This view is in sharp contrast to Erinosho's (1979) picture of modern psychiatric care in Nigeria. This author states that currently at least two major orientations, both of which recognize the importance of traditional healing, are crystallizing among Nigerian psychiatrists. The "non-culture-bound" treatment approach recognizes the role of native healers by incorporating discussion of rituals in psychotherapy. Erinosho (1979, p. 1574) gives the example of treatment of members of the Yoruba group, all of whom are generally familiar with diagnostic procedures of native healers and the use of herbs and symbolic rituals in dealing with mental illness: "For the most patients and nonpatients, such treatment is seen to entail accepted rituals that are meant to placate or destroy diabolical spiritual forces. Group psychotherapy for Yoruba patients is dominated by patients' verbalizations of the evil forces that lie behind their illness." He states that psychiatrists sharing this orientation recognize the importance of these rituals in individual psychotherapy but do not encourage their patients to undertake them. The second orientation—the "culture-bound" approach, not only acknowledges the role of rituals, but "emphasizes a convergence of healing methods through the joint role of native healers and western-oriented psychiatrists or treatment techniques in the therapetuc process" (Erinosho, 1979, p. 1574).

Use of Traditional Healing
in Western Therapy

Unlike the integrative culture-bound therapy of Nigeria described by Erinosho (1979), most Western therapies appear to use folk healing as an ancillary mode for education, and to a lesser degree for treatment. There is no evidence of a syncretic or organically evolved system of merging traditional and psychodynamic or behavioral approaches. Nevertheless, the past decade has seen the development of folk healing usage on various levels. These include a number of quasi-syncretic approaches and even ritual simulations that, although contrived, appear to be useful in alleviating distress. Delgado (1979) has suggested five types of involvement of folk healers in mental health programs: (1) training of professionals; (2) consultee-centered consultation; (3) referral agent; (4) reciprocal arrangement for referrals; and (5) a cotherapeutic relationship, with the healer physically present in the mental health setting as an equal therapist. Ruiz and Langrod's (1976) description of the levels of their actual involvement with *espiritistas* have included (a) identification of mediums in the program; (b) visits to spiritual centers and observations of their *modus operandi*; (c) exchange of views with mediums; (d) reciprocal referrals; (e) research for training non-Hispanic staff; and (f) plans for share-training workshops.

In this schema, the folk healing is not actually done in the community mental center and is not part of its formal program. Rather, folk healers have a consultant, training, and mutual-referral role. This role has not been reported in a number of different mental health facilities in the United States. An initiator in this area has been the Lincoln Community Mental Health Center in New York (Ruiz & Langrod, 1976). A major research effort, the Inner-City Support Systems Project in Newark, New Jersey, directed by anthropologist Vivian Garrison (1977, 1978), has studied and conferred with both Afro-American (Walton & Curet, 1979) and Hispanic (Rodriguez & Hernandez, 1979) folk healers. A consultant, training, and referral role for *curanderos* has been reported in the Pilsen CMHC in Chicago (Weclew, 1975). Medicine men have been involved for many years in treatment of Navajo Indians (Bergman, 1973) and for Eskimo villagers (Attneave, 1974) as part of the Indian Health Service (see Dinges, Trimble, Manson, & Pasquale, 1981, for brief overview).

In the Therapist-Spiritist Training Project in Puerto Rico (Koss, 1980), spiritist healers, mental health workers, and medical and other health professionals have met on neutral academic ground for over three ten-month periods to exchange ideas and discuss cases. Therapists and spiritists have begun to refer patients (sometimes themselves) to each other. One of the goals of the project is to develop new psychotherapeutic approaches from a synthesis of the most effective healing techniques.

Beginning with Weidman's (1978) work on alternate healing systems, the University of Miami's New Horizons CMHC has used folk healers for consultant, training, and referral purposes (including espiritistas, *santeros*, Haitian *houngans* or *mambos*, and Black American root doctors), and has also done some quasi-syncretic interventions, performed by knowledgeable staff of appropriate cultural background.

TABLE 6.1
Folk Healing in U.S. Mental Health Systems: Empirical Levels of Application

	Folk Healer	*Mental Health Practitioners*
Education[a]	key informant role	formal education of peers or students (cultural training)
	formal education of mental health practitioner (cultural training)	
Referral	reciprocal, primarily as target	reciprocal, primarily as source
Practice	individual case consultation	use of folk healer information with clients (checklist, feedback, loop), maintaining "scientific" modern approach
	Autonomous practitioner role (auxiliary status to mental health practitioner	dual-therapist role-modern and traditional modes
	autonomous practitioner role (parallel status to mental health practitioner)	ritual healing (simulation) ritual healing (quasi-syncretic)
	collaborative role as cotherapist	collaborative role as cotherapist

a. In the main, the educational variable has been unidirectional, that is, folk healers have educated mental health practitioners, while mental health practitioners, using anthropological literature and knowledge from key informants, have educated their peers in aspects of patient care related to ritual belief systems. A suggested mode, however, is for reciprocal education, so that folk healers may use their status and prestige to educate their communities in those preventive stategies that are sanactioned by the mental health system and that are not alien to the culture.

THE PROFESSIONAL AS KNOWLEDGEABLE ABOUT FOLK BELIEFS

As an authority on Afrocuban *santeria*, Sandoval (1977, 1979) uses her knowledge of the *santos* (patron gods) to communicate to patients her understanding of their belief system, particularly in their attributions of cause and blame. This knowledge is used (a) to establish trust and rapport, (b) to reinforce the credibility of the therapist, (c) to legitimize the therapist's authority to stop antisocial behavior, and (d) to use the patient's own symbolic system in interpretation. As an example of the third use noted above, the exhortation to an acting-out patient that "your *santo* doesn't want you to make a scandal!" has immediately stopped aversive behavior. As an example of the last use, the patient's products, such as painting or dreams, can be interpreted within the spiritist belief system.

Sandoval (personal communication, 1981) has pointed out that while Western therapists can use the symbolic system and learn how to communicate in the idiom of the patient, performance of an intervention in the folk healing mode can cause role ambiguity. The intrinsic ambivalence of this role places the professional at a disadvantage with colleagues and folk healers as well, and may cause unwarranted client expectations. The mediation and interpretation function is more appropriate for the Western professional.

Leininger (1978), also, in her work with Spanish-speaking families of schizophrenic daughters believed to be bewitched, has demonstrated that a skillful therapist may enable family members to ventilate their feelings about witchcraft without actually entering the magical system. In the process, expression of interpersonal fears and hostilities, and insight into acculturational stresses and conflicts, permits dynamic change and an increase in group unity.

The Professional as Folk Healer

An example of simulated ritual healing is given by Kreisman (1975), who describes two cases of integrated *curanderismo* with psychotic Mexican-American patients. These involved a prescribed regimen of prayer, isolation, and personal deprivation, together with "a curandero's herb," which were actually doxepin hydrochloride (Sinequan). Kreisman (1975, p. 83) has himself questioned the ethics of this role, but has equated it with that of the "general practitioner offering subtherapetuc doses of a minor tranquilizer to his somatizing patient together with strong incantations that the medication will cure him."

In the dual-therapist role, components of folk healing as integrated with accepted psychological or psychiatric treatment. This method does not fuse two belief systems, but rather uses them in tandem. One intervention focuses on removing the source of bewitchment, since without this, the patient cannot begin to be helped. The other intervention is geared toward adapting patient or family behavior that generates or reinforces the presumed victimization by a malevolent other. An example of this approach is an intervention by Bestman (Bestman, Lefley, & Scott, 1976), in which a young Black American girl suffering from fainting spells because of visitations from a dead cousin's spirit was given instructions on how to remove the spirit (wearing a cross, placing money in the four corners of the room), while behavior modification techniques were taught to members of the extended family.

There are several other instances in the New Horizons CMHC in which a mental health practitioner of similar cultural background to the patient, and knowledgeable about rituals, has actually performed a cleansing or exorcism with documented positive effects. These include several cases of syncretic Afro-American and Caribbean rituals performed by an ordained minister of Bahamian birth, Reverend Philip Clarke, who is also coordinator of the New Horizons Bahamian team. Merging herbs, oils, "grave dirt," and proper incantation with biblical numerology, Clarke was able to help "rooted" patients who could not be helped by other means. One patient who had required psyciatric hospitalization every August for the last four years was able to go for a year without an episode.

Another example was an exorcism for a hospitalized Haitian schizophrenic patient. Performed by Haitian mental health technicians, this was the closest to a truly syncretic ritual, since it merged masonic rites with those of *Vodun*. This ceremony observably calmed a floridly psychotic patient and permitted earlier discharge than had been anticipated.

Collaborative Therapy:
Professionals and Folk Healers

Sandoval (1977, p. 62) has suggested a model for collaborative treatment as follows:

> If *santeros* and professionals could collaborate, the professional "caring for the mind" could take a leading role in the professional development aspects of the treatment; while the *santero* could complement this by offering what he can do best; intensive support, opportunity to socialize in an accepting group, and brokerage for obtaining the backing of "supernatural power" in "caring for the soul."

In a later article (Sandoval, 1979, p. 147), a patient's words confirm the validity of this model and suggest that there is little or no perceived dissonance in being the recipient of two therapeutic approches:

Both the social wokers and the *santera* help me solve my personal problems. The social worker is a person just like me [who] knows how to control me so that I will control myself. She works with my mind, she is like my physician. She works inside of me mentally. She speaks to me and gives me [motivation], makes me reason. . . . My *santera* makes available to me a strength and power which is greater than me. She gives me firmness and security that I can do things. My *santera* . . . controls my guardian angel . . . controls the invisible spirits which get attached to me and cause evilness.

These comments focus on the benefits derived by the patient from the two systems. The nature of the collaborative relationship among the providers, however, seems problematic. While Koss (1980) suggests that a certain amount of sharing of diagnostic and therapeutic technology is feasible in spiritist-psychiatrist interaction, Dinges et al. (1981), in an excellent discussion of the cross-cultural communication pitfalls, state that most working relationships with American Indian traditional healers have ended in failure.

Attitudes Toward an Integrated System

The attitudes of Western professionals seem bipolar on the subject of folk healing. On the one hand, the entire thrust of Western philosophy, including the premises underlying psychotherapeutic care, appear to militate against the magical causal explanations and the ritual remedies of folk healing. On the other hand, many Western therapists, particularly those dissatisfied with the limited outcomes of their interventions, seem to veer toward consultation with folk healers. There is some indication that social scientists place greater value on folk interventions than do community members or newly trained indigenous professionals (Gaviria & Stern, 1980). There is also some indication that proponents of the newer, existential therapies in the West tend to glorify alternate states of consciousness asssociated with native healing. Essentially, however, it would seem that Western psychiatric practice should be antagonistic to folk healing in its conceptualizations of etiology, function, and therapeutic goals. Modern psychiatry focuses on an internal locus of control of reinforcement, while folk healing perceives mental distress as externally controlled. Sandoval (1977, 1979), however, has added greatly to our understanding by pointing out how supernatural belief systems

TABLE 6.2

Comparison of Western and Traditional Mental Health Treatment Approaches

Dimension	Western Mental Health Systems	Folk Healing
Etiology		
Source	biogenetic/psychosocial/interactional	supernatural/interpersonal/interactional
Time focus	typically historical	typically ahistorical
Precipitating factors	psychosocial—— interpersonal—— intrapsychic	supernatural—— interpersonal
Locus of control	internal	external
Diagnosis		
Techniques	observation, interview, history, testing	observation, interview, divination
Symptomatology	manifest ——(may or may not specify)—— latent (intrapsychic)	manifest ——(specifies)—— latent (supernatural)
Treatment		
Techniques	psychodynamic: diffuse, may ignore presenting complaint; focuses on underlying psychodynamics	therapeutic regime specific to presenting complaint; focuses on counteracting etiologic agent, sometimes changing behavioral contingencies to avoid recurrence
	behaviorist: specific to presenting complaint; focuses on changing contingencies of reinforcement directive, nondirective	directive
Therapeutic mode of interaction	therapist-patient communication	therapist communication with supernatural agents
Patient involvement	primarily verbal	primarily ritualistic

functionally permit mastery through manipulation of the powerful gods.

In certain respects, the community mental health rationale moves toward a closer accommodation with folk concepts than the psychoanalytic notion of ultimate human rationality and change. The individualistic ethos holds that humans are the masters of their own destinies if they can learn to respond correctly to adverse events and to prevent their recurrence in their own lives and those of their children. Community mental health approaches, subsuming those of social psychiatry and community psychology, postulates externally controlled sources of distress—economic, political, sociocultural— that may require massive social interventions, as well as individual environmental manipulations, to ultimately provide surcease. While the sociocultural view may be far removed philosophically from the view of the world as a magical and frightening place in which the supernatural must be unceasingly propitiated, the notion of external forces, environmental manipulation, and systemic change (an alteration in relationships and vectors), is common to both. More important, however, is the community mental health movement's ideological recognition of the need for cultural definitions of etiology, symptomatology, and treatment of mental disorder.

Sympathetic professionals have also admired the fact that spiritual healers not only accomplish what they themselves cannot—such as propitiation, cleansing, and removal of a hex—but the healers can often do better what psychotherapists try to do. Ruiz and Langrod (1976), for example, note that spiritualists can provide avenues for acting out forbidden wishes; favor abreaction through practice of rituals; and increase self-esteem by providing group support (see also Garrison, 1978). Sandoval (1977) has pointed out that *santeria* offers believers a guilt-releasing set of beliefs as well as mechanisms for controlling one's fate.

The recognition of folk healing as a therapeutic tool, however, seems to rest less on its Western-sanctioned legitimacy than on its patent benefits to the believer patient on several counts: (a) as an explanatory device for his or her misery; (b) as a participatory vehicle for attaining relief; (c) as a group support system; and (d) as a preventive mechanism that offers recognition of potentially noxious stimuli. Further, the collaborative model outlined here is one indicator of how compartmentalized healing may actually lead to the patient's perception of a more holistic result.

SUMMARY AND CONCLUDING REMARKS

In this chapter, discussion of mental health service delivery has involved a cross-cultural perspective that is essentially bilateral. Unicultural and cross-cultural research, particularly in developing countries, sheds light on what is peculiarly value bound or nonadaptive in Western conceptualizations of prevention, diagnosis, and treatment. Conversely, with planning under way to transplant the community mental health model to developing countries, it becomes important to address some empirical deficits of this model that have emerged during its developmental history in the West.

Major areas of concern include the scope of mental health services and appropriate target groups; service priorities and how they articulate with undeserved populations; the prevention/treatment ratio; governance, planning, coordination, and locus of decision making; accountability; and integration of mental health services with other human services, particularly with the general health delivery system.

The growth of human services ideology and the movement toward deinstitutionalization have often led to competing demands for scarce resources. For this reason, this chapter has tended to emphasize service delivery to the severely psychiatrically disabled, specifically the chronic patient. Because of their high visibility and disruptive potential, the severely disordered are generally the first population to require Western modes of intervention; but history shows that this is also the group most likely to be swept further back on the high waves of community mental health ideology.

A number of findings from various directions in unicultural and cross-cultural research suggest that there may be viable alternatives to hospitalization and, indeed, alternatives to a lifetime of chronicity and dysfunction. The findings of the International Pilot Study of Schizophrenia suggest that support and stress may be key variables in the continuation of illness. There are several foci in the new approaches to service delivery that seem to be relevant cross-culturally. The following are now viewed as legitimate components of comprehensive mental health systems:

(1) an integrated, wide-spectrum approach with social, medical, and environmental interventions;
(2) ecological therapeutic approaches and network building;
(3) for deinstitutionalized patients, case management and community support services as essential components of aftercare; and
(4) where feasible, an integration of indigenous healing approaches with Western medical/psychiatric systems.

REFERENCES

Abad, V., Ramos, J., & Boyce, E. (1974) A model for delivery of mental health services to Spanish-speaking minorities. *American Journal of Orthopsychiatry, 44*, 548-595.

Acosta, F. X., & Sheehan, J. G. (1978). Self-disclosure in relation to psychotherapist expertise and ethnicity. *American Journal of Community Psychology, 6*, 545-553.

Alcohol, Drug Abuse, and Mental Health Administration [ADAMHA]. (1981). Italian psychiatric services undergo national change. *ADAMHA News, 7*(10).

Andrulis, D. P. (1977). Ethnicity as a variable in the utilization and referral patterns of a comprehensive mental health center. *Journal of Community Psychology, 5*, 231-237.

Anthony, W. A. (1977). *The principles of psychiatric rehabilitation.* Amherst, MA: Human Resource Development Press.

Anthony, W. A., et al. (1972). Efficacy of psychiatric rehabilitation. *Psychological Bulletin, 78*, 447-456.

Appleton, W. S. (1974). Mistreatment of patients' families by psychiatrists. *American Journal of Psychiatry, 131*, 655-657.

Arey, S., & Wahrheit, G. J. (1980). Psychosocial costs of living with psychologically disturbed family members. In L. N. Robins, P. J. Clayton, & J. K. Wing (Eds.), *The social consequences of psychiatric illness* (pp. 158-175). New York: Brunner/Mazel.

Attneave, C. (1974). Medicine men and psychiatrists in the Indian Health Service. *Psychiatric Annals, 4*(1), 49-55.

Bachrach, L. L. (1978). A conceptual approach to deinstitutionalization. *Hospital and Community Psychiatry, 29*, 573-578.

Beels, C. C., & McFarlane, W. R. (1982). Family treatments of schizophrenia: Background and state of the art. *Hospital and Community Psychiatry, 33,* 541-550.

Bergman, R. L. (1973). A school of medicine men. *American Journal of Psychiatry, 130,* 663-666.

Bestman, E. W., Lefley, H. P., & Scott, C. S. (1976, March). *Culturally appropriate interventions: Paradigms and pitfalls.* Paper presented at the 53rd Annual Meeting of the American Orthopsychiatric Association, Atlanta, GA.

Borus, J. F., Burns, B. J., Jacobson, A. M., Macht, L. B., Morrill, R. G., & Wilson, E. M. (1980). *Coordinated mental health care in neighborhood health centers* (National Institute of Mental Health Series DN No. 3, DHHS Publication No. ADM 80-996). Washington, DC: Government Printing Office.

Brenner, M. H. (1973). *Mental illness and the economy.* Cambridge, MA: Harvard University Press.

Brown, G. W., Birley, J. L., & Wing, J. K. (1972). Influence of family life on the course of schizophrenic disorders. A replication. *British Journal of Psychiatry, 121,* 241-258.

Budson, R. D. (1979). Sheltered housing for the mentally ill: An overview. *McLean Hospital Journal, 4*(3), 140-157.

Caplan, G. (1964). *Principles of preventive psychiatry.* New York: Basic Books.

Carkhuff, R., & Pierce, R. (1967). Differential effects of therapist race and social class upon patient depth of self-exploration in the initial clinical interview. *Journal of Consulting Psychology, 31,* 632-634.

Carpenter, M. D. (1978). Residential placement for the chronic psychiatric patient: A review and evaluation of the literature. *Schizophrenia Bulletin, 4,* 384-398.

Carstairs, G. M. P(1973). Psychiatric problems in developing countries. *British Journal of Psychiatry, 123,* 271-277.

Collomb, H. (1978). L'economie des villages psychiatriques. *Social Science and Medicine, 12C,* 113-115.

Committee on Psychiatry and the Community. (1978). *The chronic mental patient in the community.* New York: Group for the Advancement of Psychiatry.

Day, R. (1982). Research on the course and outcome of schizophrenia in traditional cultures: Some potential implications for psychiatry in the developed countries. In M. J. Goldstein (Ed.), *Preventive intervention in schizophrenia: Are we ready?* (DHHS Publication No. ADM 82-1111). Washington, DC: Government Printing Office.

De Hoyes, A., & De Hoyes, G. (1965). Symptomatology differentials between Negro and white schizophrenics. *International Journal of Social Psychiatry, 11,* 245-255.

Delgado, M. (1979). Therapy Latino style: Implications for psychiatric care. *Perspectives in Psychiatric Care, 17*(3), 107-115.

Delgado, M., & Scott, J. F. (1979). Strategic interventions: A mental health program for the Hispanic community. *Journal of Community Psychology, 7,* 187-197.

Dinges, N. G., Trimble, J. E., Manson, S. M., & Pasquale, F. L. (1981). Counseling and psychotherapy with American Indians and Alaskan natives. In A. J. Marsella & P. Pedersen (Eds.), *Cross-cultural counseling and psychotherapy.* Elmsford: NY: Pergamon.

Dohrenwend, B. P., Dohrenwend, B. S., Gould, M. S., Link, B., Neugenbauer, R., & Wunsch-Hitzig, R. (1980). *Mental illness in the United States.* New York: Praeger.

Doi, T. (1969). Japanese psychology, dependency need, and mental health. In W. Caudill & Tsung-Yi (Eds.), *Mental health research in Asia and the Pacific.* Honolulu: East-West Center Press.

Doi, T. (1973). *The anatomy of dependence.* New York: Jodansha International.

Draguns, J. G. (1981). Cross-cultural counseling and psychotherapy: History, issues, current status. In A. J. Marsella & P. B. Pedersen (Eds.), *Cross-cultural counseling and psychotherapy.* Elmsford, NY: Pergamon.

Egeland, J. A. (1978). *Ethnic value orientation analysis: A research component of the Miami Health Ecology Project* (Vol. 2). Miami: University of Miami School of Medicine.

Eisenberg, C. (1980). Honduras: Mental health awareness changes a community. *World Health Forum,* 1(1,2), 72-77.

Erinosho, O. A. (1979). The evolution of modern psychiatric care in Nigeria. *American Journal of Psychiatry, 136,* 1572-1575.

Fairweather, G. W. (Ed.). (1980). *The Fairweather Lodge: A twenty-five year perspective.* San Francisco: Jossey-Bass.

Fields, S. (1974). Foster communities for the mentally ill. *Innovation,* pp. 3-16.

Garrison, V. (1977). Doctor, *espiritista,* or psychiatrist? Health seeking behavior in a Puerto Rican neighborhood of New York City. *Medical Anthropology, 1*(2), 65-191.

Garrison, V. (1978). Support systems of schizophrenic and nonschizophrenic Puerto Rican migrant women in New York city. *Schizophrenia Bulletin, 4,* 561-596.

Gaviria, M., & Stern, G. (1980). Problems in designing and implementing culturally relevant mental health services for Latinos in the U.S. *Social Science and Medicine, 14B,* 65-71.

Gittelman, M. (1978). Needed: Long term care in the community. *International Journal of Mental Health, 6*(4), 3-8.

Gittelman, M., Dubuis, J., & Gillet, M. (1973). Recent developments in French public mental health. *Psychiatric Quarterly, 47,* 509-520.

Glasscote, R. (1975). The future of the community mental health center. *Psychiatric Annals, 5*(9), 382-387.

Goffman, E. (1962). *Asylums: Essays on the social situations of mental patients and other inmates.* Chicago: Aldine.

Goldman, H. H. (1982). Mental illness and family burden: A public health perspective. *Hospital and Community Psychiatry, 33,* 557-559.

Goldstein, M. J. (1981). Editor's notes. In M. J. Goldstein (Ed.), *New developments in interventions with families of schizophrenics.* San Francisco: Jossey-Bass.

Guthrie, G. M. (1966). Structure of maternal attitudes in two cultures. *Journal of Psychology, 62,* 155-165.

Gynther, M. D. (1972). DIFFS in norms: White norms and black MMPI's: A prescription for discrimination? *Psychological Bulletin, 78*(5), 386-402.

Haase, H. J. (1981). Follow up treatment and aftercare of discharged schizophrenic patients. *Schizophrenia Bulletin, 6,* 619-626.

Harding, T. W. (1975). Mental health services in the developing countries: The issues involved. In T.A. Baasher, G. M. Carstairs, R. Giel, & F. R. Hassler (Eds.), *Mental health services in the developing countries.* Geneva: World Health Organization.

Hatfield, A. B. (1978). Psychological costs of schizophrenia to the family. *Social Work, 23,* 355-359.

Higginbotham, H. N. (1976). A conceptual model for the delivery of psychological services in non-Western settings. In R. Brislin (Ed.), *Topics in culture learning* (Vol. 4). Honolulu: East-West Center Press.

Higginbotham, H. N. (1979). *Delivery of mental health services in three developing Asian nations: Feasibility and cultural sensitivity of "modern psychiatry."* Unpublished doctoral dissertation, University of Hawaii.

Hogarty, G. E. (1971). The plight of schizophrenics in modern treatment programs. *Hospital and Community Psychiatry, 22,* 197-203.

Holdstock, T. L. (1979). Indigenous healing in South Africa: A neglected potential. *South African Journal of Psychology, 9,* 118-124.

Hollingshead, A. B., & Redlich, F. C. (1958). *Social class and mental illness.* New York: John Wiley.

Hsu, F. L. (1972). American core value and national character. In F. L. Hsu (Ed.), *Psychological anthropology* (rev. ed.). Cambridge, MA: Schenkman.

Jegende, R. O. (1981). A study of the role of socio-cultural factors in the treatment of mental illness in Nigeria. *social Science and Medicine, 15A,* 49-54.

Jenkins, J. H. (1981, December 3). *The course of schizophrenia among Mexican Americans.* Paper presented at the annual meeting of the American Anthropological Association, Los Angeles.

Kapur, R. (1979). The role of traditional healers in mental health care in rural India. *Social Science and Medicine, 13B,* 27-31.

Karno, M. (1982, October 16). *The experience of schizophrenia in Mexican American Families.* Paper presented at the meeting of the Society for the Study of Psychiatry and Culture, San Miguel Regla, Mexico.

Kirk, S. A., & Therrien, M. E. (1975). Community mental health myths and the fate of former hospitalized patients. *Psychiatry, 38,* 209-217.

Kluckhohn, F. R., & Strodtbeck, F. L. (1961). *Variations in value orientations.* New York: Harper & Row.

Korer, J. R., Freeman, H. L., & Cheadle, A. J. (1978). The social situation of schizophrenic patients living in the community. *International Journal of Mental Health, 6*(4), 45-65.

Koss, J. D. (1980). The Therapist-Spiritist Training Project in Puerto Rico: An experiment to relate the traditional healing system to the public health system. *Social Science and Medicine, 14B,* 255-266.

Kreisman, J. J. (1975). The *curandero's* apprentice: A therapeutic integration of folk and medical healing. *American Journal of Psychiatry, 132,* 81-83.

Kringlen, E. (1981). Schizophrenia research in the Nordic countries. *Schizophrenia Bulletin, 6,* 579-585.

Lamb, H. R. (1977). Rehabilitation in community mental health. *Community Mental Health Review, 2*(4), 1-8.

Lamb, H. R., & Oliphant, E. (1978). Schizophrenia through the eyes of families. *Hospital and Community Psychiatry, 29,* 803-806.

Lamb, H. R., et al. (Eds.). (1976). *Community survival for long-term patients.* San Francisco: Jossey-Bass.

Lambo, T. A. (1966). Patterns of psychiatric care in developing African countries: The Nigerian program. In H. R. David (Ed.). *International trends in mental health.* New York: McGraw-Hill.

Lambo, T. A. (1978). Psychotherapy in Africa. *Human Nature, 1,* 32-39.

Lebra, W. P. (Ed.). (1976). *Culture-bound syndromes, ethnopsychiatry, and alternate therapies.* Honolulu: University Press of Hawaii.

Lefley, H. P. (1972). Modal personality in the Bahamas. *Journal of Cross-Cultural Psychology, 3,* 135-147.

Lefley, H. P. (1974, April). *Ethnic patients and Anglo healers: An overview of the problem in mental health care.* Paper presented at the Ninth Annual Meeting of the Southern Anthropological Society, Blackburg, VA.

Lefley, H. P. (1975a, February). *Dependency in cross-cultural perspective.* Paper presented at the annual meeting of the Society for Cross-Cultural Research, Chicago.

Lefley, H. P. (1975b). Approaches to community mental health: The Miami model. *Psychiatric Annals, 5*(8), 26-32.

Lefley, H. P. (1976). Acculturation, child rearing and self esteem in two North American Indian tribes. *Ethos.*

Lefley, H. P. (1979a). Prevalence of potential falling-out cases among the Black, Latin and non-Latin white populations of the city of Miami. *Social Science and Medicine, 13B*(2). 113-114.

Lefley, H. P. (1979b). Environmental interventions and therapeutic outcome. *Hospital and Community Psychiatry, 30,* 341-343.

Lefley, H. P., & Bestman, E. W. (1982). Community mental health and minorities: A multi-ethnic approach. In S. Sue & T. Moore (Eds.), *Community mental health in a pluralistic society.* New York: Human Sciences Press.

Lenininger, M. (1978). *Transcultural nursing: Concepts, theories, and practices.* New York: John Wiley.

Levy, L., & Rowitz, L.(1973). *The ecology of mental disorder.* New York: Behavioral Publications.

Lombillo, J. R., & Geraghty, M. (1973, April). *Ethnic accountability in mental health programs for Mexican-American communities.* Paper presented at the annual meeting of the Society for Applied Anthropology, Tucson, AZ.

Marcos, L., & Alpert, M. (1976). Strategies and risks in psychotherapy with bilingual patients. *American Journal of Psychiatry, 133,* 1275-1278.

Mehryar, A., & Khajavi, F. (1974). Some implications of a community mental health model for developing countries. *International Journal of Social Psychiatry, 21,* 45-52.

Miller, F. T., Mazade, N. A., Muller, S., & Andrulis, D. (1978). Trends in community mental health programming. *American Journal of Community Psychology, 6,* 191-198.

Miranda, M. (Ed.). (1976). *Psychotherapy for the Spanish-speaking*. Los Angeles: Spanish-Speaking Mental Health Research Center.

Mollica, R. F., & Redlich, F. (1980). Equity and changing patient characteristics—1960 to 1975. *Archives of General Psychiatry, 37*, 1257-1263.

Mosher, L. R., & Keith, S. J. (1981). Psychosocial treatment: Individual, groups, family and community support approaches. In *Special report: Schizophrenia, 1980* (DHHS Publication No. ADM 81-1064). Washington, DC: Government Printing Office.

Munoz, R. F. (1976). The primary prevention of psychological problems. *Community Mental Health Review, 1*(6), 5-15.

Padilla, A. M. (1981). Pluralistic counseling and psychotherapy for Hispanic Americans. In A. J. Marsella & P. Pedersen (Eds.), *Cross-cultural counseling and psychotherapy* (pp. 195-227). Elmsford, NY: Pergamon.

Papajohn, J., & Spiegel, J. (1975). *Transactions in families*. San Francisco: Jossey-Bass.

Pepper, B., Kirshner, M. C., & Ryglewicz, H. (1981). The young adult chronic patient: Overview of a population. *Hospital and Community Psychiatry, 32*, 463-469.

Peszke, M. A., & Winthrob, R. (1974). Emergency commitment: A transcultural study. *American Journal of Psychiatry, 131* 36-40.

Phillips, H. P. (1965). *Thai peasant personality*. Berkeley: University of California Press.

Pines, A., & Maslach, C. (1978). Characteristics of staff burnout in mental health settings. *Hospital and Community Psychiatry, 29*, 233-237.

President's Commission on Mental Health. (1978). Report of the Task Panel on Deinstitutionalization, Rehabilitation and Long Term Care. In *Task panel reports submitted to the President's Commission on Mental Health* (Vol. 2, pp. 356-375). Washington, DC: Government Printing Office.

Rodriguez, P., & Hernandez, A. (1979, March). *Healers in the Hispanic communities: Possibilities for consultation programs*. Paper prepared for the annual meeting of the Society for Applied Anthropology, Philadelphia.

Ross, H. K. (1975). Low-income elderly in inner-city trailer parks. *Psychiatric Annals, 5*(8), 86-90.

Ruiz, P. (1977). Culture and mental health: A Hispanic perspective. *Journal of Contemporary Psychotherapy, 9*, 24-27.

Ruiz, P., & Langrod, J. (1976). The role of folk healers in community mental health services. *Community Mental Health Journal, 12*, 392-398.

Ruiz, P., Vazquez, W., & Vazquez, K. (1973). The mobile unit: A new approach in mental health. *Community Mental Health Journal, 9*, 18-24.

Sandoval, M. C. (1977). Santeria: Afrocuban concepts of disease and its treatment in Miami. *Journal of Operational Psychiatry, 8*(2), 52-63.

Sandoval, M. C. (1979). Santeria as a mental health care system: An historical overview. *Social Science and Medicine, 13B*, 137-151.

Sandoval, M. C., & Tozo, L. (1975). An emergent Cuban community. *Psychiatric Annals, 5*(8), 48-63.

Sartorius, N., Jablensky, A., & Shapiro, R. (1978). Cross-cultural differences in the short term prognosis of schizophrenic psychosis. *Schizophrenia Bulletin, 4,* 102-113.

Schizophrenia Bulletin. (1981). 7(1).

Schulberg, H. C. (1977). Community mental health and human services. *Community Mental Health Review, 2*(6), 1-9.

Sidel, R., & Sidel, V. (1972). The human services in China. *Social Policy,* pp. 25-34.

Simon, R., et al. (1973). Depression and schizophrenia in hospitalized black and white mental patients. *Archives of General Psychiatry, 28,* 509-512.

Snyder, P. (1981). Ethnicity and folk healing in Honolulu, Hawaii. *Social Science and Medicine, 15B,* 125-132.

Soni, S., Soni, S. D., & Freeman, H. L. (1978). Group homes for psychiatric patients: An evaluation of six years' experience in the domestic resettlement of chronic psychiatric patients. *International Journal of Mental Health, 6(4), 66-79.*

Spiegel, J. P. (1981). Hispanic training for non-Hispanic mental health professionals. *World Journal of Psychosynthesis, 13,* 25-30.

Sue, S. (1977). Community mental health services to minority groups. *American Psychologist, 32,* 616-624.

Szapocznik, J., Kurtines, W., & Fernandez, T. (1980). Bicultural involvement and adjustment in Hispanic-American youths. *International Journal of Intercultural Relations, 4,* 353-365.

Szapocznik, J., Scopetta, M., & King, O. E. (1978). Theory and practice in matching treatment to the characteristics of Cuban immigrants. *Journal of Community Psychology, 6,* 112-122.

Szasz, T. (1974). *The myth of mental illness.* New York: Harper & Row.

Talbott, J. A. (1981). The emerging crisis in chronic care. *Hospital and Community Psychiatry, 32,* 447.

Thomas, A., & Sillen, S. (1972). *Racism and psychiatry.* New York: Brunner/Mazel.

Uyanga, J. (1979). The characteristics of patients of spiritual healing homes and traditional doctors in Southeastern Nigeria. *Social Science and Medicine, 13A,* 323-329.

Vaughn, C. E., & Leff, J. P. (1976). The influence of family and social factors in the course of psychiatric illness: A comparison of schizophrenic and depressed neurotic patients. *British Journal of Psychiatry, 129,* 125-137.

Walton, D., & Curet, E. (1979, March). *Afro-American folk healers and mental health care.* Paper prepared for the annual meeting of the Society for Applied Anthropology, Philadelphia.

Waxler, N. E. (1974). Culture and mental illness: A social labeling perspective. *Journal of Nervous and Mental Disease, 159,* 379-395.

Waxler, N. E. (1979). Is outcome for schizophrenia better in nonindustrial societies? The case of Sri Lanka. *Journal of Nervous and Mental Disease, 167,* 144-158.

Weclew, R. V. (1975). The nature, prevalence and level of awareness of "curanderismo" and some of its implications for community mental health. *Community Mental Health Journal, 11,* 145-154.

Weidman, H. H. (1973). *Implications of the culture broker concept for the delivery of health care.* Paper presented at the annual meeting of the Southern Anthropological Society, Wrightsville Beach, NC.

Weidman, H. H. (1975). Concepts as strategies for change. *Psychiatric Annals, 5*(9), 17-19.

Weidman, H. H. (1978). *Miami Health Ecology Project report: A statement on ethnicity and health* (Vol. 1). Miami: University of Miami School of Medicine.

Weidman, H. H. (1979). Falling out: A diagnostic and treatment problem viewed from a transcultural perspective. *Social Science and Medicine, 13B,* 95-112.

Westermeyer, J., & Pattison, E. M . (1981). Social networks and mental illness in a peasant society. *Schizophrenia Bulletin, 7,* 125-134.

Wing, J. K. (1975, October). *Planning and evaluating services for chronically handicapped psychiatric patients in the U.K.* Paper presented at a conference on Alternatives to Mental Hospital Treatment, Madison, WI.

Wing, J. K. (1980). Social psychiatry in the United Kingdom: The approach to schizophrenia. *Schizophrenia Bulletin, 6,* 556-565.

Woodbury, M. A. (1969). Community-centered psychiatric intervention. *American Journal of Psychiatry, 125,* 619-625.

II: Culture-Specific Applications

7

TRADITIONAL ASIAN MEDICINE
Applications to Psychiatric Services in Developing Nations

ANTHONY J. MARSELLA
HOWARD N. HIGGINBOTHAM

WESTERN RATIONALISM AND MENTAL HEALTH

The concept of "mental health" is not unique to the Western world. It has long been a part of the cultural traditions of many Asian cultures under the rubric of religious and healing systems that emphasize harmonious relations among body, mind, and spirit. However, it has been mainly within the Western cultural traditions that these three levels of functioning have been separated and individually institutionalized via distinct professional roles, knowledge systems, and physical facilities (see Figure 7.1). To a large extent, this separation has been part of the legacy of Western scientific and technological ideologies that began in the eighteenth century to secularize a heretofore religiously inspired discourse about madness (see Foucault, 1971).

We, the inheritors of Western scientific rationalism, are today faced with a rather interesting dilemma. Clearly, the concept of "mental health" has become a valued goal. We frequently find ourselves speaking of "healthy values," "healthy relationships," and "healthy behavior." Yet, we seem to be somewhat confused about what these things actually mean. There seems to be an awareness that somehow mental health involves harmonious relationships among all levels of our functioning, and certainly between the individual and the world about him or her. Yet we seem unable to attain this harmony. To a certain extent, this appears to be due to the tremendous discontinuities fostered by our continually changing technological developments, which outpace our capacity to establish meaningful linkages

Institutional Representations

		Roles	Facilities	Knowledge
	Body	Physicians Physical and Biological Scientists Nurses	Hospitals Clinics Laboratories	Medicine Physiology Anatomy Chemistry
Levels of Human Functioning	Mind	Mental Health Professionals	Hospitals Clinics Rest Homes Laboratories	Psychology Theology Psychiatry
	Spirit	Priests Ministers Psychics	Churches Temples Shrines	Philosophy Theology Mysticism

Figure 7.1   Institutionalizing the Separation of Body, Mind and Spirit: The Legacy of Western Science and Philosophy

between our world and our experience. We are, in the industrialized West, forced to deal with life in small pieces without access to the beliefs and philosophies that permit some semblance of a holistic perspective to emerge and thrive.

This dilemma is particularly cogent to those of us whose notions of personhood derive from the "disenchanted" or empiricist world view associated with the Protestant Reformation in Europe (Gaines, 1982). The second great tradition in the West, that of Mediterranean Europe and Catholicism, in contrast, permits the intersection of spiritual and mundane realms. Gaines (1982, p. 180) found that the latter Western tradition embraced the "belief in a magical, enchanted world wherein threads of this world and those of the world beyond are woven together in a single fabric of perception and experience as in the medieval (e.g., Latin) world view."

But, in spite of the many limitations and inadequacies that characterize Western empiricist approaches to mental health, we have not been hesitant to import it to non-Western cultural milieus. Every day, Western mental health concepts, methods, facility designs, and professional training techniques are being fostered, encouraged, and promoted as the answer to the non-Western world's mental health

problems, regardless of the many pernicious effects[1] (see Higginbotham, in press).

The purpose of this chapter is to discuss the possibility of applying
traditional Asian healing systems to the mental health problems of
developing Asian nations. Our major argument is that psychiatric
services in developing Asian nations could greatly benefit from the
integration of traditional Asian healing systems with the existing
Western systems that have been established in recent years. Further,
we argue that this integration can and should occur at all levels,
including basic philosophy, problem conceptualization, treatment,
prevention, and facility design. The chapter is divided into three
sections: The first concerns problems in establishing Western mental
health services in Asian nations; the second addresses applications of
traditional Asian healing systems; and the third discusses the
implementation of traditional Asian healing systems.

PROBLEMS IN ESTABLISHING
MENTAL HEALTH SERVICES IN ASIA

Administrative Problems

A number of people have written about the many administrative
problems in establishing mental health care in Asian nations (for
example, see Carstairs, 1973; Giel & Harding, 1976; Higginbotham,
in press; Neki, 1973a, 1973b; Sartorius, 1977; World Health
Organization, 1975a, 1975b). These sources have pointed out that
there are many problems confronting the development of modernized
psychiatric services in developing countries, including the following:
(1) low national priorities for health and particularly for mental
health; (2) limited institutional and organizational support networks;
and (3) trained human resource shortages and difficulties. Let us
examine these problems more closely.

Clearly, in nations with low capital resources, the priorities for
health are often placed behind those for defense and agricultural and
industrial development (see Harding, 1975; Neki, 1973a, 1973b;
World Health Organization, 1978). Further, when health is able to
receive a portion of a nation's resources, those resources usually
must be directed toward infectious diseases, nutritional programs,
sanitation, and other more publicly focused problems. Mental health

funds are almost always limited to maintenance of custodial-care institutions (Higginbotham, in press).

Health planning bodies are often more responsive to political pressures than to health needs. This means that mental health planning and legislation are often ignored or relegated to low-priority positions within the total political process. Further, within this context, Higginbotham (in press) has pointed out that psychiatric health care services become eliminated from the entire network of governmental and social processes that are needed to initiate and sustain a mental health care system. For example, Higginbotham has noted that weak national health leadership hinders (1) the creation of legislation for strengthening and regulating psychiatric services; (2) the recruitment and effective use of qualified health human resources; (3) the coordination of educational efforts with community and governmental health needs; (4) the establishment of national and regional health service systems; (5) the development of health insurance plans incorporating mental health care; (6) the absence of need assessment and program evaluation mechanisms; and (7) the biased distribution of the minimal mental health resources that are available in favor of urban-educated elite. Kiernan (1976) points out that the majority of mental health services in developing countries are directed toward the urban residents, who constitute only a small portion of the populations of those countries.

Another problem in the development of mental health services is the lack of human resources (Higginbotham, in press; Sartorius, 1977; World Health Organization, 1975a, 1975b). Few individuals enter the mental health professions largely because mental health training programs for psychiatry, social work, psychology, and psychiatric nursing are neither prestigious nor well developed. Further, there is a growing awareness among interested individuals that working conditions are poor and that status and pay are low. Carstairs (1975) points out that there is also a tendency for other medical specialties to look down on the psychiatric professions. The shortage of human resources is also compounded by the fact that individuals interested in pursuing mental health careers often travel abroad for their education and then return with technical competencies that are not applicable to the local situations (that is, if they choose to return at all).

In addition to the many public administrative problems that curtail the establishment of mental health services in developing Asian nations, there are also a number of problems related to the cultural relevance of the services that are provided.

Cultural-Relevance Problems

For those mental health professionals who are dedicated to the development of "modernized"[2] psychiatric services, there is yet another set of problems that they must encounter, stemming from the cultural relevance of the services they seek to provide. Though one cannot question the commitment and sense of mission that characterize these leaders, there is a substantive basis for questioning the particular choice of service delivery models they seek to implement, specifically psychiatric models embodying assumptions, concepts, and methods that have little meaning for cultures with profoundly different traditions.

In the last half century, as part of the continuing effect of the colonial and neocolonial heritage, it has become the accepted practice for mental health professionals in developing countries to model their services after those in the West. In the immediacy of their desire to adapt Western technology, they have come to ignore the fact that large buildings, sizable staffs, and extensive treatment alternatives do not make a meaningful or effective mental health service system. What many of these pioneers have forgotten is that for a healing system to be effective, it must be acceptable; and acceptability is a function of the attributes that users assign to the system. What has been ignored is the rather simple fact that the introduction of a mental health delivery system based on alien cultural premises and traditions represents a major social change process that is subject to the same resistances that are true of other social changes. It is obvious to every religious missionary that religious conversion takes a great deal of time and requires a systematic penetration of the culture of the future converts. Further, it is clear that the final form the religion will assume in the activities of the convert is often a synthesis of new and old, rather than an unconditional acceptance of the new. This is because many aspects of the cultural milieu in which the convert lives have no continuity with the new religion. This rather simple example of the acceptability of a social change highlights the problems faced by the introduction of a Westernized psychiatric service to non-Western people. Let us examine these problems more closely.

Physical Locations

The actual physical locations of the mental health services for either acute or chronic care are most often centered in urban settings that are inaccessible to the majority of a country's population, especially the rural poor. Thus, even though people may be aware of institutional care, they are unlikely to use it because of the travel cost and time required to reach urban destinations.

Lack of Support Networks

Because the mental health service network is poorly developed and frequently not integrated with primary care or primary prevention services, those problems for which patients desire professional consultation may become quite chronic and debilitating. This makes treatment difficult and increases the chance of failure.

Diagnostic Bias

When patients do come for care, their problems are often classified in Western diagnostic terms. Most often, biomedical nosologies have little relevance for the patient and his or her immediate kin group, who typically assume responsibility for managing illness episodes (Kleinman, 1980). Further, the conceptualization of the problem in terms of Western biologic and psychologic assumptions of causality is largely discordant with popularly held folk theories based upon such notions as supernatural intervention, fate, and cosmological harmony (see Marsella & White, 1982).

Communication Problems

The mental health professionals involved with the patient may be either Western or ruling-class nationals who have been trained in the West, and thus are unable to communicate effectively with the patient on either a verbal or a nonverbal level. In addition, in some Asian countries, there is distinct social stratification according to economic position, geography, and subcultural membership. These groups are often in conflict with one another, yet it is possible that the mental health system may force one group to be treated by another. In other words, there is often a failure to have cultural, social class, and regional group representation in the administration of a mental health system.

Treatment Bias

Treatment in many mental health centers has become almost exclusively based on medications. These medications may be useful in either lowering or raising a level of arousal, but they fail to address the full spectrum of causes that may be implicated in the etiology, maintenance, and enhancement of the problem. In addition, the reliance solely on medication ignores the healing potential that is present in a closer, more ritualized healer-patient relationship in which there is extensive involvement with the patient, the patient's family, and the patient's environment. Even such potentially powerful sources of placebo effects as touching, holding, chanting, and specific behavioral commands are ignored. As Kleinman and Sung (1976, pp. 55-56) have pointed out, under the above circumstances disease may be dealt with, but healing does not necessarily occur:

> Healing is not so much a result of the healer's efforts [as it is] a condition of experiencing illness and care within the cultural context of the health care system. Healing is a necessary activity that occurs to the patient, and his family and social nexus, regardless of whether the patient's disorder is affected or not. The health care system provides psychosocial and cultural treatment . . . for the illness by naming and ordering the experience of illness, providing meaning for that experience, and treating the personal, family, and social problems which comprise the illness, and thus it heals, even if it is unable to effectively treat the disease.

Treatment Errors

Mental health professionals working in Asia will make mistakes in diagnosis if they lack familiarity with the cultural setting in which the patient's problems develop and remain ignorant of the discourse strategies underpinning effective communication in the indigenous language environment (Gumprez, 1982). This can result in faulty, ineffectual, or even harmful treatment. For example, the first author's extensive research program on ethnocentric aspects of depressive experience and disorder (see Marsella, 1980) has revealed numerous ethnocultural variations in the manifestation (Marsella, Kinzie, & Gordon, 1973), experience (Tanaka-Matsumi & Marsella, 1976), measurement (Marsella, Sanborn, Kameoka, Brennan, & Shizuru, 1975), and personality correlates (Yanagida & Marsella, 1978) of depression.

Although there may be cultural invariances in certain patterns of disorder, there is a growing body of research that is pointing out the critical role of cultural factors across all clinical parameters, including etiology, expression, disability, course, and outcome (for example, see Draguns, 1980; Marsella, 1979, 1980; Fabrega, 1972; Waxler, 1974; Sartorius, Jablensky, & Shapiro, 1978). Indeed, it is our opinion that all mental disorders are "culture-specific" disorders and that this term should not be reserved for the so-called exotic syndromes, such as *latah, koro, imu, susto, mali-mali,* and so forth (see Marsella & White, 1982).

Iatrogenic Problems

Mental health professionals frequently produce many iatrogenic effects in the course of their treatments. These iatrogenic problems are related to both the medications and the difficulties created by giving advice or counseling that is at variance with the patient's cultural milieu (Higginbotham, 1979a). Without being aware of it, deviance may be fostered or stress added to the patient's life by encouraging behavior patterns that are at odds with the social nexus in which the patient resides. There is also an increased chance of iatrogenic problems developing because of the absence of extensive follow-up care networks in which the patient's progress and response to medication can be monitored effectively.

Stigma

Psychiatric care is highly stigmatized. To admit that a problem of madness exists evokes the possibility of witchcraft, evil, family curses, sorcery, and other supernatural explanations (see Asuni, 1975; Connor, 1982; Higginbotham, in press; Lieban, 1967). This problem is faced in dealing with indigenous healers as well; however, the risks of institutionalization and the permanent loss of a family member are minimized. In our experience in Sarawak, the Philippines, and Thailand, once patients came to the hospital, they were at risk of being abandoned by their families and never returning home. This obviously makes for a great deal of resistance to seeking psychiatric care from Western-trained mental health professionals.

These eight problems regarding the cultural relevancy of developing Westernized psychiatric systems to serve non-Western populations are only a few of the many problems that must be dealt with by mental health professionals. Good psychiatric care requires extensive sensitivity to the cultural traditions of the people who are served.

Clearly, it would be unfair and inaccurate to state that indigenous healers do not have problems treating patients. They also have their share of failures and for many of the same reasons. But the notion that indigenous healers are "quacks" and "frauds" and that only Western ("modern") approaches to mental health care are valid is the greater inaccuracy. The argument that Western approaches are scientifically based while indigenous or traditional approaches are based on magic and superstition is invalid because it mistakes technology for science and because it assumes that only "rational" thinking guides Western assumptions and techniques. Further, it ignores centuries of effective healing knowledge.

In brief, the major point of this section has been to discuss both the administrative and the cultural-relevance problems that confront efforts to establish a Western-based psychiatric service in developing Asian nations. As should be clear, the problems are numerous and the solutions may reside in our ability to bring about a synthesis between Asian and Western philosophies and treatment approaches within the context of the same mental health system. This alternative offers a number of valuable options for strengthening and expanding existing services and for increasing the "acceptability" of the current psychiatric services.

SOME APPLICATIONS OF
TRADITIONAL ASIAN HEALING SYSTEMS

The scope of traditional Asian healing systems is quite broad and encompasses everything from naturalistic to supernaturalistic assumptions and therapeutic methods. A review of these systems is beyond the scope of this chapter and the interested reader is encouraged to pursue the topic in greater depth through publications in medical anthropology, Asian philosophy, and ethnomedicine (for example, see Fabrega, 1971, 1972; Kao & Kao, 1979; Kleinman, Kunstader, Alexander, & Gale, 1975; Lieban, 1973; Lock, 1980; Mulholland, 1979; Nakamura, 1964; Reid, 1979). However, it is important for us to acknowledge that traditional Asian healing systems are very sophisticated with regard to their assumptions about the nature of health and disorder and the treatments necessary for cure and prevention.

It is unfortunate that Western biomedical systems, especially those related to mental health, have tended to ignore traditional Asian healing approaches or to limit their interest to purely academic levels of inquiry and debate. Fortunately, the dissatisfaction with Western medicine in both the East and the West and the growing consumer demand for a more meaningful medical care system may force Western medical professionals to implement alternative healing philosophies and methods. Today, consumers of medical services are calling for greater accountability from professionals. They are seeking more than technical care and expertise—they are asking for a quality of care that encompasses all levels of functioning: holistic care (see La Patra, 1978). Many traditional Asian healing systems have long been based on philosophies and methods that emphasize "holistic" care.

Philosophical Applications

Contemporary Western medical systems are evidencing a growing disenchantment with the older "germ" and "mechanistic" models of health and disease. An outcome of this disenchantment has been the emergence of a number of alternative medical systems, including stress theory, general systems theory, holistic medicine, behavioral medicine, and various public health approaches. Further, another sign of this discontent is the growing attraction of various "Eastern" approaches to health care, including acupuncture, massage therapies, meditation, holistic diet/exercise activities, and herbal medicines. Thus it may be an opportune time for Western medical systems to shed their unwarranted sense of superiority and apply some traditional Asian philosophies that are very congruent with the new Western approaches.

For example, many traditional Asian healing systems are based on the ancient Chinese world view of "man as a microcosm," a reflection of the entire cosmic process and structure (Lock, 1980). Needham (1962, p. 281) writes:

> Things behaved in particular ways not necessarily because of prior actions or impulsations or other things, but because their position in the ever-moving cyclical universe was such that they were endowed intrinsic natures which made that behavior inevitable for them. If they did not behave in those particular ways they would lose their relational position in the whole (which made them what they were), and turn into something other than themselves. They were thus parts in existential dependence upon the whole world organism. And they reacted upon one another.

These thoughts are part of ancient Chinese philosophy, but they sound amazingly similar to contemporary Western notions in field theory physics, theoretical biology, and organismic psychology.

Within the context of such a philosophy, disorder, whether physical or mental, is viewed as a dysfunction in relationship. As Lock (1976, pp. 15-17) observes:

> Sickness ... is not seen so much in terms of an intruding agent, although this aspect of disease causation is acknowledged, but rather due to a pattern of causes leading to disharmony. These causes can be environmental, social, psychological, or physiological level. ... The function of diagnosis is not to categorize a patient as having a specific disease, but to record the total body state and its relationship to the macrocosm of both society and nature as fully as possible. ... the model allows explanations for the benefit of the patient to be in broad psycho/social and environmental terms which are readily understandable and cognitively acceptable. These explanations can be used by the patient to account for the occurrence of suffering in the context of his or her own life history at that moment. ... Therapy is designed to act on the whole body—removal of the main symptoms is not considered adequate as all parts of the body are thought to be interdependent—in this sense the model is holistic. ... It is believed that the functioning of man's mind and body is inseparable.

A similar philosophy is found in the ancient Indian traditions. Kitaeff (1976, pp. 2-8), in a paper on the healing traditions of India, Nepal, and Tibet, noted the individual, social, and spiritual focus of the Indian tradition:

This total cultural continuity of individual, community, and god, and of sickness, health, and ultimate liberation involves the whole spectrum of the healing process—the purification of body, speech, and mind. Precise correspondence exists among all these elements, so that the elementary substances in the body are considered a microcosm of divine forces in the universe and the yogic or tantric ceremonies of healing may simultaneously act upon the physical and subtle bodies to achieve spiritual wholeness as well as physical and mental well-being. . . . Like Greek and Egyptian medicine, Indian and Tibetan medicine had a divine origin: as part of the universal creation of Brahma, the science of Ayurveda was handed down through the god Indra for the relief of suffering mankind. Since then, religious elements have been inseparable from all aspects of study and practice. . . . Not only the study of a new medical test, but also the giving and taking of medicine are accompanied by prayers. . . . Methods of treatment are different for the systems of Ayurvedic, yogic, and ceremonial or tantric medicine, but all share the common object of achieving universal wholeness and harmony through natural principles.

It is readily apparent that whether one is speaking of ancient Chinese or ancient Indian healing traditions, the emphasis is on the treatment of the whole person—holistic care. This approach may well be the most valuable for defining true mental health, a point that more and more Western approaches are beginning to recognize. The holistic nature of the Asian healing philosophies may be the most meaningful direction for the Western approaches to follow.

Many Western psychiatric approaches seem either unwilling or unable to offer the patient the hope of a new lifestyle or a new behavior pattern. They are content with symptom control at the expense of stupor and side effects. They are oriented toward the molecular at the expense of the molar, toward the part at the expense of the whole, toward the "disease" at the expense of the "illness."

Kleinman and Sung (1976, p. 4) state:

Let us call *disease* any primary malfunctioning in biological and psychological processes. And, let us call *illness* the secondary psychosocial and cultural responses to disease, e.g., how the patient, his family, and social network react to his disease. Ideally, clinical care should treat both disease and illness. Up until several decades ago, when their ability to control sickness began to increase dramatically, physicians were interested in treating both disease and illness. At present, however, modern professional health care tends to treat disease but not illness; whereas, in general, indigenous systems of healing tend to treat illness, but not disease.

Thus what we are advocating is that Western psychiatric healing systems begin actively to integrate Asian healing philosophies into their approaches. This practice would have beneficial effects for everyone and especially for Asian patients, because the healing services would be more continuous with their cultural traditions.

Now let us turn to possible Asian healing methods that might be effectively implemented by Western psychiatric healing systems.

Healing Method Applications

The spectrum of methods used in traditional Asian healing procedures is far beyond the scope of the present chapter. Thus we will only offer general comments. As is true of Western medicine, Asian healing systems make use of drugs from natural sources, diet, exercises, various forms of meditation and body control, counseling and advice, massages, and spiritual practices. There are numerous sources that provide overviews of these methods (see Jaggi, 1973; Jocano, 1973; Kiev, 1964; La Patra, 1978; Lebra, 1976; Leslie, 1976; Lieban, 1973; Marsella & White, 1982; Rechung, 1973; Reynolds, 1976; Wallnofer & von Rottauscher, 1974).

The study of ethnobotany has revealed that many traditional cultures have made sophisticated use of various plants and herbs for healing. A well-known example of this is the famed "snakesroot" of ancient India, which contains rauwolfia alkaloids that have powerful tranquilizing effects. This is only one example of hundreds of substances that have been used with success in traditional Asian healing. Kitaeff (1976, pp. 8-9) states that Indian physicians use a number of substances:

Traditional Indian physicians have used medicines derived from vegetables, animals, and earth. Almost every part of plants can be used as drugs, but the time and method of collecting the plant products for medicinal purposes is an art that requires training and experience to know the proper seasons, places, and signs of full growth. . . . Medicines can be administered in many different forms—as decoctions, powders, pills, syrups, medicinal wine, oily or ash-like medicine. They act on the body through the influence of their *rasa* (taste), *vipaka* (post-digestive content), *virya* (potency), and *prabhava* (special action).

There is certainly every reason to believe that traditional medicines may have a meaningful role in dealing with various psychiatric problems, especially when considered against the numerous side effects and iatrogenic effects that are part of the use of Western medicines.

In addition to plant and herbal medicines, the use of diet therapies is something that could be assiduously applied by traditional healers working in Western psychiatric settings. The use of various physical therapies, such as massages, saunas, Tai Chi Chuan, Aikido, yoga, polarity therapy, and acupuncture, is also something that should be explored. At the present time, Western psychiatric approaches are devoid of touch, manipulation, and patient activity. For the most part, drugs are prescribed and the patient is simply left alone to let the drugs do their work. It is exciting to envision a psychiatric setting where many of the previously cited Asian healing methods would be available for the patient.

Although counseling and psychotherapy assume many different forms in both the East and the West, it is clear that more could be done with various forms of hypnosis, meditation, palmistry, astrology, and general advice and counseling. Japanese culture has two culturally derived systems of psychotherapy (Morita therapy and Naikan therapy) that might be valuably adapted for other Asian cultural settings.

Closely allied to the various psychotherapy approaches are the numerous traditional Asian healers who emphasize spiritual approaches, including mediums, shamans, mystics, and masseurs. One wonders what improvements might occur in Western psychiatric settings if such practitioners were to establish true healing centers, offering their patients a spectrum of healing methods in which the patient could find knowledge, health, and enlightenment. How sterile our current hospitals and clinics are by comparison. We offer many drugs, a few words, and an occasional pat on the back. Can we really expect mental health to develop in such a situation? There is no vitality, no energy, no hope! Is it any wonder that non-Western patients tend to avoid these places except as a last resort? And often, when patients do come, they fail to return. There is no meaning in the treatment they receive and, without meaning, the source of healing is often lost.

Thus what we are advocating is a healing community, where the emphasis is on providing the patient accessibliity to a spectrum of healing method directed not toward control, or even toward mental health—the harmonious relationship of body, mind, and spirit. Such centers could be termed "holistic healing centers" or "omnibus healing centers" rather than "hospitals" or "clinics." They could be centers for prevention as well as acute care; centers for learning, not solely for treatment. The only places we know of that even come close to such facilities are the "Esalen"-type programs, Hindu-inspired ashrams or residential-spiritual centers now present in several Western cities, and Lambo's treatment center in Nigeria, in which traditional healers and psychiatric professionals work in a residential treatment center surrounded by a patient community (Lambo, 1966). As is well known, Lambo's center provides for care of the patient by relatives living in a village close to the hospital. Treatment includes traditional methods such as confession, dances, rituals, and herbs; the indigenous healer is an active part of the treatment strategy. All of this has produced less stigma for the patient and more effective care.

Although the specific procedures that would be necessary for effective patient care in such a setting are more complex, they are not beyond possibility. It is true that there would be risks of conflicts between competing systems and personnel, but these could be worked out, especially in an atmosphere of mutual respect. We predict that many of the administrative problems that would inevitably arise would come from the chauvinistic attitudes of the Western-trained personnel rather than from the traditional healers. But it would be possible to alter these attitudes through effective training and administrative procedures. Some of the steps in establishing such a system are described in the next section.

TOWARD A SYNTHESIS OF TRADITIONAL ASIAN MEDICINE AND CONTEMPORARY WESTERN PSYCHIATRIC CARE SYSTEMS

Recently the senior author codirected a government-funded training program to develop effective cross-cultural counselors and psychotherapists (see Marsella & Pedersen, 1981). What became quite clear in the course of this program was that teaching therapists to work with patients from different cultural traditions is a Brobdingnagian task that goes far beyond the mere exchange of academic knowledge about cultural differences. There is a need for information about specific cultural practices and forms, but there is also a more important need to sensitize trainees to both their own cultural assumptions and the cultural phenomenology of the patients with whom they will be dealing. We would suggest the following steps toward a synthesis of the different healing traditions.

Cultural Awareness

Perhaps the most important step in the successful synthesis of the diverse healing traditions is an awareness of the role of culture in human behavior. Though everyone acknowledges cultural differences, a true awareness and grasp of the enormous role that culture plays in our lives eludes most people's understanding. This is especially true of health care professionals, who are socialized to look on all patients as the same because of obvious physical similarities or diagnostic grouping. But few people are actually sensitive to the fact that culture guides and channels our basic epsitemology, our sense of time, space, and causality. Indeed, all of our notions about health and disorder are culturally and linguistically determined (see Good & Good, 1982). Yet we continue to train therapists who are oblivious to the phenomenological perspectives of the patients they treat and to their own cultural biases. Professionalism diminishes the therapist's capacity to respond emphatically to culturally divergent clients and replaces experiential awareness with stereotypic judgments. Therefore, we suggest that the first step be extensive training in culture awareness. We should train healers, Eastern and Western, to be aware of culture—their own as well as that of others. As part of this training, it would be very useful to encourage an awareness of the different healing systems as cultures in and of themselves. This might reduce chauvinism.

In addition to teaching about the culture of medicine, efforts should also be made to teach healers about the culture of *being* a patient. They should learn about "sick roles," "healing roles," and "medical sociology." This learning should occur at an *experiential* level through the many culture-learning exercises that have been developed. Following training in culture awareness, training can then be focused on an awareness of the ethnocultural traditions of the patients the healers will treat.

Awareness of Patient's Cultural Traditions

Culture influences all aspects of functioning, from the physiological to the spiritual. This influence is extended not solely through basic values and beliefs, but also through the food people eat and the environments in which they live. If we are truly to understand behavior, whether it be adaptive or dysfunctional, we must understand its cultural foundations. Thus a second step in the synthesis is to teach an awareness of the patient's culture.

Our personal experience in "culture learning" has led us to believe that a number of instructional methods must be used in teaching about a cultural tradition. These methods involve experiential, didactic, and analogue approaches. There are facts to be learned, but there are also feelings to be experienced. Brislin (1979) provides a good overview of these alternative culture orientation approaches.

Assessment of the Cultural Accommodation of the Service Delivery System

A third step toward successful synthesis of the different healing traditions is an assessment of the Western psychiatric system's willingness to adjust to and be sensitive to the patient's cultural traditions. Perhaps the most extensive work in this area has been conducted by Higginbotham (1979b, in press). He investigated the mental health delivery system of seven Asian countries with regard to their "accommodation" to patient cultural traditions via an elaborate scale. This scale permitted him to assess the different points of bias, including conceptions of disorder, treatment preferences, staff attitudes toward patients, and so forth. Higginbotham's Ethnotherapy and Culture Accommodation Methodology is useful in appraising a system's cultural biases.

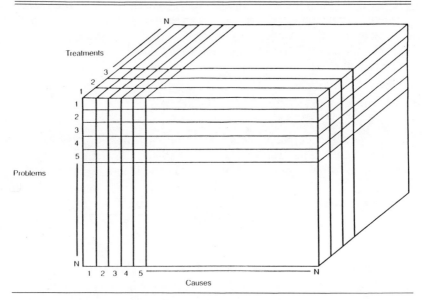

Figure 7.2   Problem, Cause, and Treatment Matrix

Development of Knowledge Regarding Patient Conceptions of Disorder, Treatment, and Causality

One of the major impediments to a successful synthesis of the different healing traditions is that Western professionals are often unaware of non-Western conceptions of disorder, treatment, and causality. In 1976, the senior author (see Marsella, 1978a, 1979, 1980) suggested that researchers initiate a series of studies on different ethnocultural groups' conceptions of disorder, treatment, and causality. He proposed the development of a series of matrices that would encompass the findings and that could be used by actual practitioners. Figure 7.2 displays a sample matrix. At the present time Marsella and his coworkers are nearing completion of a matrix study on Japanese, Chinese, Samoan, Hawaiian, and Korean people. This study has revealed that each group has a very distinct series of conceptions of disorder, treatment, and causality. The findings should prove useful to hospital and clinic staff, who often tend to be insensitive to the cultural variations of their patients.

Use of Non-Western Healers
in Western Health Settings

No synthesis of the different healing traditions can occur unless Western professionals are willing to accept and respect the fact that there are indigenous healers who have as much if not more legitimacy as they have in caring for the mental health problems of non-Wesern people. As La Patra's (1978) recent book demonstrates, even the older medical establishment in the West is under fire to broaden its perspective by including new healing alternatives. Given this fact, it should not be too difficult for Western psychiatric systems in non-Western countries to broaden their perspectives by including non-Western healers as coworkers in the common effort to promote better mental health. Naturally, clinical settings must adopt policies and allocate resources toward the replications of indigenous healing conditions to ensure that folk healers are not stripped of their therapeutic potency when collaborating within institutional milieus. As noted previously, Lambo's work in Nigeria (see Lambo, 1966; see also Collomb, 1973) is a visible testimony to the success of such an approach.

Alteration of Western Concepts
of Mental Health

The last step we wish to propose toward the synthesis of Western psychiatric services and traditional Asian medicine is the alteration of existing Western conceptions of mental health in favor of the more holistic approaches characteristic of Asian healing traditions. As was noted previously, both the East Asian and the Indian traditions emphasize the harmony among physical, mental, and spiritual levels of functioning. In contrast, Western biomedical approaches to mental health tend to separate these levels. Often medications alone are provided, or psychotherapy may be used without attention to physiological functioning. And, of course, the more spiritual aspects of being (that is, those concerned with mystical and transcendental experiences) are usually ignored or relegated to the religious community. Clearly, human beings function at many different levels. Mental health, as the traditions of Asia have long recognized, requires attention at all of these levels. It is time for the West to recognize this basic truth.

NOTES

1. Western approaches to mental health care should not be considered totally useless and destructive. The major problem appears to be the fact that our philosophies and methods have become disengaged from a meaningful perspective. We speak of mental health, but give people pills. When we provide psychological therapies, we do so in isolation from the everyday life of the person, ignoring the many social and community influences that help maintain behavior. We have confused cure with control and, in the process, our patients continue to feel isolated and estranged from their own experience.

2. It is unfortunate that many people have confused modernization with Westernization. The two are very different. It is clear that our contemporary world, our "modern" world, have not necessarily progressed through adoption of Western cultural traditions. Progress may well require that the Western world reconsider many aspects of its functioning, especially with regard to humanistic concerns. Western cultural traditions and economic practices are rapidly producing a broad array of social problems that may now be beyond solution. A more thorough discussion of this point is available in Marsella (1978a).

REFERENCES

Asuni, T. (1975). Existing concepts of mental illness is different cultures and different forms of treatment. In T. Baasher, G. Carstairs, R. Giel, & F. Hassler (Eds.), *Mental health services in developing countries*. Geneva: World Health Organization.

Baasher, T. (1975). Principles of psychiatric care. In T. Baasher, G. Carstairs, R. Giel, & F. Hassler (Eds.), *Mental health services in developing countries*. Geneva: World Health Organization.

Brislin, R. (1979). Cross-cultural orientation programs. In A. J. Marella, R. Tharp, & T. Ciborowski (Eds.), *Perspectives on cross-cultural psychology*. New York: Academic Press.

Carstairs, M. (1973) Psychiatric problems of developing countries. *British Journal of Psychiatry*, 271-277.

Carstairs, M. (1975). Psychiatry in basic medical education. In T. Baasher, G. Carstairs, R. Giel, & F. Hassler (Eds.), *Mental health in developing countries*. Geneva: World Health Organization.

Collomb, H. (1973). The meeting of two systems of patient care with regard to the treatment of mental illness in Africa. *Social Science and Medicine, 7,* 623-633.

Connor, L. H. (1982). The unbounded self: Balinese therapy in theory and practice. In A. J. Maresella & G. M. White (Eds.), *Cultural conceptions of mental health and therapy*. Dordrecht, Netherlands: Reidel.

Draguns, J. (1980). Psychopathology. In H. Triandis & J. Draguns (Eds.), *Handbook of cross-cultural psychology: Vol. 6. Psychopathology.* Boston: Allyn & Bacon.

Fabrega, H. (1971). Medical anthropology. In B. Siegal (Ed.), *Biennial review of anthropology.* Palo Alto, CA: Stanford University Press.

Fabrega, H. (1972). The study of disease in relation to culture. *Behavioral Science, 17,* 183-203.

Foucault, M. (1971). *Madness and civilization: A history of insanity in the Age of Reason.* London: Tavistock.

Gaines, A. D. (1982). Cultural definitions, behavior and the person in American psychiatry. In A. J. Marsella & G. M. White (Eds.), *Cultural conceptions of mental health and therapy.* Dordrecht, Netherlands: Reidel.

Giel, R., & Harding T. (1976).Psychiatric priorities in developing countries. *British Journal of Psychiatry, 128,* 513-522.

Good, B., & Good, M.J.D. (1982). Toward a meaning centered analysis of popular illness categories: "Fright illness" and "heart distress" in Iran. In A. J. Marsella & G. M. White (Eds.), *Cultural conceptions of mental health and therapy.* Dordrecht, Netherlands: Reidel.

Gumprez, J. J. (1982). *Discourse strategies: A study of interactional sociolinguistics.* Cambridge: Cambridge University Press.

Harding, T. (1975). Mental health services in developing countries: Some issues involved. In T. A. Baasher, G. M. Carstairs, R. Giel, & F. Hassler (Eds.) *Mental health services in developing countries.* Geneva: World Health Organization.

Higginbotham, H. (1979a). Cultural issues in providing psychological services for foreign students in the United States. *International Journal of Intercultural Relations, 3,* 49-85.

Higginbotham, H. (1979b). Culture and delivery of psychological services in developing nations. *Transcultural Psychiatric Research Review, 16,* 7-27.

Higginbotham, H. (in press). *Third World challenge to psychiatry: Culture accomodation and mental health care.* Honolulu: University Press of Hawaii.

Jaggi, O. P. (1973). *History of science and technology in India.* New Delhi: Atma Ram and Sons.

Jocano, F. ((1973) *Folk medicine in a Phillippine municipality.* Manila: National Museum.

Kao, M. & Kao, A. (Eds.). (1979).*New medicine* New York: Neale Watson.

Kiernan, W. (1976). *Strengthening of mental health services in Thailand.* Geneva: Mental Health Division.

Kiev, A. (Ed.). (1964). *Magic, faith, and healing.* New York: Free Press.

Kitaeff, R. (1976). *The healing spectrum in India, Nepal, and Tibet.* Paper presented at the International Conference on Religion and Parapsychology. Tokyo.

Kleinman, A., Kunstader, P., Alexander, E., & Gale, J. (EDS.). (1975). *Comparative studies of health care in Chinese and other societies.* Washington, DC: Government Printing Office.

Kleinman, A. (1980).*Patients and healers in the context of culture.* Berkeley: University of California Press.

Kleinman, A., & Sung, B. (1976). *Why do indigenous practitioners successfuly heal?* Paper presented at the conference on The Healing Process, Michigan State University, East Lansing.

Lambo, T. (1966). Patterns of psychiatric care in developing African countries: The Nigerian village program. In D. David (Ed.), *International treads in mental health.* New York: McGraw-Hill.

La Patra, J. (1978). *Healing: The coming revolution in holistic medicine.* New York: McGraw-Hill.

Lebra, W. (Ed.). (1976). *Culture-bound syndromes, ethnopsychiatry, and alternative therapies.* Honolulu: University Press of Hawaii.

Leslie, C. (Ed.). (1976). *Asian medical systems.* Berkeley: University of California Press.

Lieban, R. (1973). Medical anthropology. In J. Honigman (Ed.), *Handbook of social and cultural anthropology.* Chicago: Rand McNally.

Lieban, R. (1967). *Cebuano sorcery.* Los Angeles: University of California Press.

Lock, M. (1976). *Oriental medicine in urban Japan.* Unpublished doctoral dissertation, University of California, Berkeley.

Lock, M. (1980). *East Asian medicine in urban Japan.* Berkeley: University of California Press, 1980.

Marsella, A. J. (1978a). The modernization of traditional cultures: Consequences for the individual. In D. Hoopes & P. Pedersen (Eds.), *Intercultural education, training, and research.* Washington, DC: Sietar.

Marsella, A. J. (1978b). Thoughts on cross-cultural studies on the epidemiology of depression. *Culture, Medicine, and Psychiatry, 2,* 343-357.

Marsella, A. J. (1979). Culture and mental disorders. In A. J. Marsella, R. Tharp, & T. Ciborowski (Eds.), *Handbook of cross-cultural psychology: Vol. 6. Psychopathology.* Boston: Allyn and Bacon.

Marsella, A. J. (1980). Depressive affect and disorder across cultures. In H. Triandis & J. Draguns (Eds.), *Handbook of cross-cultural psychology: Vol. 6. Psychopathology.* Boston: Allyn and Bacon.

Marsella, A. J., Kinzie, D., & Gordon, P. (1973). Ethnic variations in the expression of depression. *Journal of Cross-Cultural Psychology, 4,* 435-438.

Marsella, A. J., & Pedersen, P. (Eds.). (1981). *Cross-cultural counseling and psychotherapy.* Elmsford, NY: Pergamon.

Marsella, A. J., Sanborn, K., Kaemeoka, B., Brennan, J., & Shizuru, L. (1975). Cross-validation of self-report measures of depression in different ethnocultural groups. *Journal of Clinical Psychology, 31,* 281-287.

Marsella, A. J., & White, G. M. (1982). *Cultural conceptions of mental health and therapy.* Boston: Reidel.

Mulholland, J. (1979). Traditional medicine in Thailand. *Hemisphere, 4,* 224-230.

Nakamura, H. (1964). *Ways of thinking of Eastern people.* Honolulu: East-West Center Press.

Needham, J. (1962). *Science and civilization in China.* Cambridge: Cambridge University Press.

Neki, J. (1973a). Psychiatry in South-East Asia. *British Journal of Psychiatry, 123,* 257-269.

Neki, J. (1973b). Psychiatric education and the social role of the psychiatrist in developing South-East Asian countries. *Social Science and Medicine, 7,* 103-107.

Rechung, R.J.K. (1973). *Tibetan medicine.* Berkeley: University of California Press.

Reid, J. (1979). Health as harmony, sickness as conflict. *Hemisphere, 4,* 194-199.

Reynolds, D. (1976). *Morita therapy.* Berkeley: University of California Press.

Sartorius, N. (1977) Compete or complement? *World Health, 12,* 28-33.

Sartorius, N., Jablensky, A., & Shapiro, R. (1978) Cross-cultural differences in the short-term prognosis of schizophrenic psychoses. *Schizophrenia Bulletin, 4,* 102-113.

Tanaka-Matsumi, F., & Marsella, A. J. (1976). Ethnocultural variations in the phenomenological experience or depression: I. Word association studies. *Journal of Cross-Cultural Psychology, 1,* 379-396.

Wallnofer, H., & von Rottauscher, A. (1974). *Chinese folk medicine.* New York: New American Library.

Waxler, N. (1974). Culture and mental illness: A social labeling perspective. *Journal of Nervous and Mental Disease, 159,* 379-399.

World Health Organization. (1975a). *Organization of mental health services in developing countries* (WHO Technical Report Series, No. 564). Geneva: Author.

World Health Organization. (1975b). *Mental health services in developing countries* (report on the Addis Adaba Conference). Geneva: Author.

World Health Organization. (1978). *Mental health in Southeast Asia Region* (report on Inter-Country Group Meeting, New Delhi, 1977). Geneva: Author.

Yanagida, E., & Marsella, A. J. (1978). Self-concept discrepancy and depression in Japanese-American women. *Journal of Clinical Psychology, 34,* 654-659.

8

AMERICAN INDIAN CONCEPTS
OF MENTAL HEALTH
Reflections and Directions

JOSEPH E. TRIMBLE
SPERO M. MANSON
NORMAN G. DINGES
BEATRICE MEDICINE

Psychopathology, mental health, and personality among North American Indians hold an enduring fascination as objects of study for social scientists. An unceasing stream of survey research findings, case studies, and critical commentary flow from researchers and practitioners. In a review of the Indian mental health literature, Attneave and Kelso (1977) remark on the overwhelming but severely imbalanced amount of available information; their review of almost 500 article represents a small portion of that literature.

Interest in Indian mental health is apparently increasing. Federal and state agencies are initiating new and presumably more culturally sensitive mental health programs. Simultaneously, research and reporting with regard to the Indian mental health "problem" is increasing. For example, recently many federal agencies developed initiatives to promote preventive intervention efforts in Indian communities (Manson, 1983). These interests and the initiatives are positive steps and have potential for improvement of mental health conditions.

In the past, most programmatic efforts to provide services in Indian mental health were guided by Euro-American psychiatric and professional traditions (see Attneave & Kelso, 1977; Trimble & Medicine, 1976). It has been demonstrated that the Euro-American tradition conflicts with the basic world view of many Indian communities. Continuation of these traditions will in all likelihood create more problems than are solved.

This chapter will explore numerous perspectives toward the phenomenon of mental health as it occurs in Indian communities. The concept of "mental health" will be examined and contrasted with certain indigenous orientations. To accomplish this, six basic tribal-specific concepts of disorder will be described. The need to formulate professional preventive mental health programs according to two (native-specific) concepts of human competence will also be discussed.

MENTAL HEALTH AS AN EVALUATIVE CONCEPT

Mental health is a concept that connotes both a particular state of professional well-being and an individual's ability to assess the state. Assessment can occur through another's inquiries into one's well-being or simply through one's awareness of the state. In fact, self-evaluation and insight coupled with the ability to do so are an integral part of mental health treatment programs—so ingrained is the assumption that few practitioners question its integrity.

The main body of mental health practitioners approach the study and treatment of mental disorders from a conventional biomedical perspective. Diagnosis and treatment are guided by the classic notion that something *in* the professional makeup of the patient is out of balance—the "in" in this case typically refers to the psyche, ego, mind, or self. Aided by the assumption that insight and catharsis promote recovery the conventional practitioner probes away with questions and suggestions. In time, if the questions are on target and the patient is accurately insightful, recovery from the disorder is imminent, if not achieved. So pervasive is the biomedical perspective that practitioners use it in a multitude of settings irrespective of the cultural, religious, and sexual orientation of the client.

Biomedical approaches to conceptualizing and treating mental disorders stem from an exclusive European and North American academic-based philosophical perspective. The person (subject) and environmental influences (objects) typically are viewed as separate from one another. In mental health settngs treatment emphasizes the person but not the environment and not the person. The many terms used in the field illustrate the embeddedness of the separateness notion: sanity and insanity, mental and behavioral disorders, psychological imbalance, self-image, deviate, personality disorders, and so on.

An abundance of evidence exists illustrating the difficulties experienced by practitioners in delivering mental health services to American Indian communities (Trimble & Medicine, 1976; Trimble, 1981; Dinges, Trimble, Manson, & Pasquale, 1981). While never quite empirically documented, one of the major problem sources could well be the way mental health, in all its facets, is conceptualized by many American Indians. Further, the separation of subject from object can be quite inconsistent with the philosophical perspectives of many North American indigenous groups—subject and object are unified and holistic in many native world views. States of mind and body, social roles, family and community organization, and the like are functionally interrelated and virtually inseparable. "Mental," "mind," "personality," and "self," for example, have unique organizing qualities within the native view. For this reason, many traditional Indians experience difficulty coming up with conceptually equivalent mental health terms in their own native languages.

American Indians, like all other linguistic groups, developed unique systems for "classifying and categorizing forms of behavior [that] fit closely within their world view and the view they have of themselves as people" (Trimble & Medicine, 1976, p. 13). In the Lakota (Sioux language), for example, "mental health" translates as *ta-un* (*being* in a state of well-being, *not a state* of well-being). Ta-un is a state of being that allows certain kinds of behavior to occur. One's ta-un is rarely if ever questioned—in fact, it's almost unthinkable to ask someone to elaborate on the state. For that matter, within many segments of the Siouan reservations, it's considered rude to inquire about a person's psychological well-being, no matter what the state of being may appear to be.

While the concept of attaining personal insight is important to many mental health intervention programs, it could also be another source of difficulty for those working with traditional Indian clients. In many Indian communities self-revelation is just not taught, revered, or in any way expected of an individual. Certainly there are ceremonial occasions in many communities where one reveals the content of dreams or vision quests; the interpretation, analysis, and insight, however, are achieved by a shaman only. Apart from ceremonial settings, private thoughts about oneself are simply kept to oneself. Thus when a mental health practitioner asks an Indian to divulge deeply held thoughts and feelings with insight and catharsis in mind, the practitioner may be asking for something that cannot be delivered.

Mental health and all of its aspects can and probably does mean quite different things to many American Indians. And the implication that mental health is grounded in different ways in the value and belief systems of one's cultural group gives rise to serious questions for cross-cultural studies of Indian mental health. The efficacy of past Indian mental health research efforts must be assessed with this implication in mind. To add further insights into the problem the following selective review of the literature on indigenous concepts of mental and behavioral disorders illustrates the often "presumptive" perspectives of many North American social and clinical scientists (see Saindon, 1933).

INDIGENOUS CONCEPTS OF DISORDER

Case descriptions, etiological theories, and discussions of native treatment approaches are largely anthropological in origin, but reflect social psychological and psychiatrist interests as well. As early as 1938, Landes (1938a p. 14) pointed out that "these descriptions afford little insight into the structure of the disorders. Hardly any attempt has been made to articulate them with the conflicts and modes of life of the people among whom they are found." The following discussion of indigenous disorders illustrates this bias. It is organized in terms of six concept areas: (1) *windigo* psychosis; (2) *pibloktoq* (arctic hysteria); (3) soul loss; (4) spirit intrusion; (5) taboo breaking; and (6) ghost sickness. The third, fourth, and fifth are drawn from Clement's (1932) broad classificatory scheme.

Windigo Psychosis

Alternately labeled *witiko* (Cooper, 1933), *wiitiko* (Parker, 1960), and *whitiko* (Bolman and Katz, 1966), windigo psychosis is characterized as symptoms of melancholia, a "craving from human flesh," and "a delusion of transformation into a witiko who has a heart of ice or who vomits ice," sometimes followed by cannibalism (Cooper, 1933, p. 20). Hallowell (1934) reported considerable variety in the clinical syndromes subsumed under this term and that, moreover, the last feature—eating human flesh—seldom if ever occurred. It has been described as a form of mental disorder, albeit a rare one, among Ojibwa, Cree, and other northern Algonkin people. Fogelson (1965) and Hay (1971) provide excellent summaries of the relevant literature.

Most descriptions of *windigo* psychosis have been abstracted from northern Algonkin folklore and mythology (Barnouw, 1963; Laidlaw, 1918, 1920, 1927; Jones, 1916). However, Teicher (1960) and Landes (1938a) offer 83 detailed case histories, the majority of which date to the middle and late 1800s. A slightly greater number of these cases involve males than females and—when age can be determined— younger as opposed to middle-aged or older adults.

Etiological questions have engendered continuing debate. Parker's (1960) psychoanalytic interpretation attributes windigo psychosis to failing ego defenses and explains subsequent behavior as an expression of conflicting dependency and aggressive needs. According to Teicher (1960, p. 113), the "conscious content of the illness, the symbols used, the delusional mold, the distortions of reality and the character of the compulsions are unmistakably dependent upon the prevailing belief system and the traditional practices within the culture." Kiev (1972, p. 84) maintains that "this is a classical depressive disorder, showing a typically prominent secondary symptom of self-depreciation and need for punishment with a culturally available explanation." He disagrees with Teicher, asserting that "there is no evidence available that the form of the illness is caused by cultural factors, nor any evidence that the Windigo belief itself has an etiological role" (Kiev, 1972, p. 85). Fogelson (1965, pp. 64-75), citing Cooper's (1933) and Landes's (1938b, p. 214) earlier observations that famine conditions, especially in the harsh subarctic regions of North America, seemed to be related to windigo psychosis, suggests the role of nutritional factors in its etiology. Rohrl (1970) explores the contribution of dietary deficiencies, specifically the lack of animal fats, and marshals an intriguing argument that references indigenous curing practices as well as previous ecological studies of ritual behavior (Rappaport, 1967). Brown (1971) takes exception to Rohrl's hypothesis, which she interprets as a primary causal factor, noting that homocide is a more likely response to individual cases than curing through nourishment alone.

Marano (1982) recently provided a critical analysis of the voluminous literature on windigo psychosis. He convincingly argues that this literature has been erected on very weak ethnographic foundation and, like a house of cards, crumbles upon close examination. Marano points out, as noted earlier in this section, that the ethnohistoric-ethnographic data actually are quite sparse, consisting of few, if any, firsthand accounts. Instead, this particular syndrome seems to have sprung from folk tales and indirect evidence that in turn gave rise to a self-perpetuating cycle of reinterpretation. Idealized accounts of the aberrant behavior *said* to be associated with windigo psychosis (notably, cannabilism) appear to have been mistakenly presumed as observable fact. Reification of this nature plagues much of what we know about other indigenously defined forms of disorder as well.

Pibloktoq

Pibloktoq, also commonly referred to as "arctic hysteria" (Foulks, 1973), is portrayed as a convulsive hysteria seizure, frequently accompanied by conversion symptoms such as limb paralysis. Wallace (1961, p. 263) offers the most comprehensive description of its manifestation:

(1) *Prodome:* In some cases a period of hours or days is reported during which the victim seems to be mildly irritable or withdrawn.

(2) *Excitement:* Suddenly, with little or no warning, the victim becomes wildly excited. He may tear off his clothing, break furniture, shout obscenely, eat feces, perform other irrational acts. Usually he finally leaves shelter and runs frantically onto tundra, or ice pack, plunges into snowdrifts, climbs onto icebergs, and may actually place himself in considerable danger, from which pursuing persons usually rescue him, however. Excitement may persist for a few minutes up to about half an hour.

(3) *Convulsions and stupor:* The excitement is succeeded by convulsive seizures in at least some cases, by collapse, and finally by stuporous sleep or coma lasting for up to twelve hours.

(4) *Recovery:* Following an attack, the victim behaves perfectly normally; there is amnesia for the experience. Some victims have repeated attacks; others are not known to have more than one.

The earlier written reports of pibloktoq include those of Dall (1870, pp. 171-72) among an Alaskan Eskimo group, Peary (1910, p. 166) during his polar expeditions, and Whitney (1911, p. 67). It has been observed primarily in arctic and subarctic Eskimo communities of North America and Greenland. Gussow (1960), Wallace (1961), and Parker (1962) review the related literature in detail.

A total of 26 case histories are available, largely in Brill (1913), Foulks (1973), Gussow (1960), and Wallace (1961). The vast majority of victims are female (21), coinciding with Peary's extended observations (compare Brill, p. 517). All are adults and, when age is mentioned, range from 20 to 52 years old. Foulks's epidemiological survey suggests that a "disproportionate number of cases tend to occur in small villages (population less than 350)."

Brill (1913) considers pibloktoq to be a form of hysteria and, citing reports of most frequent occurrence among women who have been abused or rebuffed by their husbands, postulates an ungratified desire for affection and tenderness as its etiological basis. Gussow (1960) concurs, adds new descriptive data, and elaborates the underlying psychodynamics. Parker (1962) extends this interpretation, linking pibloktoq to permissive Eskimo child-rearing practices, their cooperative social organization and communalistic value system, and the socially sanctioned outlets for hostility as well as hysterialike behavior role models in traditional Eskimo religion. Freeman, Foulks, and Freeman (1978, p. 203), considering only North Alaskan males, deem the hysteria to be an acute dissociative reaction, "precipitated by separation or loss of the object, in an individual who has not been able to complete the psychological processes of 'separation-individuation' in childhood, and is not able to deal with threatened or actual object' loss." Thus they too seek its explanation in terms of early socialization and psychodynamic constructs such as dependency and frustration. However, Leighton (1961) cautions:

> It is hard to assess the significance of "hysteria" as a diagnosis since it is influenced by the frequency of disturbances in women, and there is a tendency in cross-cultural psychiatry to interpret as hysterical any unusual or bizarre symptomology if duration and intensity do not justify a label of schizophrenia. (compare Boag, 1970, p. 116).

Wallace and Ackerman (1960) reinforce this point and call for an interdisciplinary study of pibloktoq that will explore alternative etiological hypotheses. Wallace (1961, p. 265) suggests, for example, that it may be related to calcium deficiency, which can:

> produce a neuromuscular syndrome known as tetany which is often complicated by emotional and cognitive disorganization. The neurological symptoms of tetany include characteristic muscular spasms of

hands, feet, throat, face and other musculature, and in severe attacks, major convulsive seizures.

Hence, earlier claims by Novakovsky (1924), Weyer, (1932, p. 386), and Jenness (1959, p. 52) that such aberrant behavior may be attributed to the prolonged darkness of the artic and severe climatic bear reexamination.

Soul Loss

Soul loss is one of five etiological concepts that Clement (1932, pp. 186-192) lists as explanations of illness among non-Western populations. The literature yields a number of case studies across diverse tribal communities in which its behavioral manifestation as an indigenous form of disorder is quite similar: specifically, sudden and repeated fainting, withdrawal, self-deprivation, and preoccupation with death and dead kindred.

Devereux (1937, p. 420) describes the Mohave *ghost-weylak* as soul loss through dream adventures that occur shortly after the death of a spouse or relative. Lacking immediate intervention, illness and death are thought to be inevitable consequences. This is reminiscent of the Seminole *soloipi:* (portion of soul residing in the heart), which also wanders in dreams, is sometimes persuaded to remain with the dead, and when absent results in illness or death (Capron, 1953; Straight, 1970). Aginsky (1940, p. 7) reports the same phenomenon among the Pomo. Here, as with the Piaute (Whiting, 1950) and Eskimo (Balikci, 1963), however, ghosts may *take* an individual's essence away, rather than coerce it. Soul loss frequently appears as an explanation of illness in ethnographies of Northwest Coast tribes, as evidenced in Murdock's (1965a, 1965b) conversations with a Tenino healer. Quoting Boas's field observations at length, Nieuwenhuis (1924, p. 355) highlights the special emphasis of the Kwakiutl, Tsimshian, and Haida: "So to all of them sickness emphasis of the Kwakiutl, Tsimshian, and Haida: "So to all of them sickness is connected either with absence of the soul or with its being weakened." *Ta watl' yesni* or "totally discouraged" among Dakota Sioux of the Standing Rock Reservation is characterized by the following:

(1) deprivation;
(2) the traveling of one's thoughts and losing one's mind to the dwelling of one's dead relatives, the ghost camp;

(3) an orientation toward the past;

(4) thoughts of death;

(5) facilitation of a process of sending one's spirits to the ghost camp by willing death, committing or threatening suicide, or drinking to excess;

(6) preoccupation with ideas of ghosts or spirits; and

(7) expression of blocked action, for example, life is hopeless (Johnson & Johnson, 1965, p. 142).

Johnson and Johnson maintain that a similar constellation of associated conditions and behaviors can be identified in anthropological records of numerous plains tribes, including the Winnebago, Cheyenne, Oglala Sioux, and Canadian Assiniboine.

Unlike the two previous concepts—and despite a rich set of case materials, mental disorder attributed to and/or labeled soul loss has not engendered much speculation about contributing factors. Aginsky (1940, p. 7) cites recurrent themes of apprehension, anxiety, and fear, but fails to explain their relationship to the cognitive and behavioral nature of this phenomenon. Johnson and Johnson (1965, p. 141) view it as a response to particularly stressful life experiences, which, in turn, gives rise to alcoholism, suicide, property destruction, child and family neglect, and social irresponsibility.

Spirit Intrusion

Spirit intrusion "includes all etiologies which hold that disease is due to the presence of evil spirits, ghosts or demons" (Clement, 1932, p. 190). Jilek and Jilek-Aal (1971, p. 1183) though referring to a specific form among Salish-speaking people of the Northwest Coast, offer an excellent profile of the general symptoms:

Comparable with those of an agitated depression, often associated with considerable somatization, hallucinatory or illusional experiences. In particular, these symptoms are: anorexia insomnia, apathy alternating with restlessness; dysphoric crying spells and nostalgic despondency; dyspnoea, precordial sensations and vague spastic pains.

Again, ethnographic accounts appear early and are frequent in number.

Hallowell (1939, 1963) depicts Ojibwa world view as an orientation toward achieving *pimadaziwin:* life, in the fullest sense of health, longevity, and freedom from misfortune. Sickness *(ackaziwin)*—of which spirit intrusion is a serious example—jeopardizes its attainment. Murdock (1965a, p. 169) discusses spirit intrusion in the context of Tenino healing practices, but does not provide sufficient case material to enable cross-tribal comparison. Among eastern subarctic Eskimo, the equivalent is *quissaatug,* "featured chiefly by compulsive passivity, withdrawal, and depression . . . accompanied by brief flurries of manic activity" (Vallee, 1966, p. 64). Jilek and Jilek-Aal (1971), Jilek and Todd (1974) , and Jilek (1974) provide records of *schwas* possession in Northwest Coast Salish communities, in which the victim has been "made sick by spirit power" (Jilek, 1974, p. 17).

Jilek (1974, p. 17) interprets *schwas* as an anomic depression, the consequences of existential frustration, discouragement, defeat, and lowered self-esteem resulting from social and cultural deprivation. In an interesting contrast, Hallowell (1963, p. 310) restates the Ojibwa explanation as follows:

> Serious cases of illness . . . are considered to be the consequence of behavior which departs from expectations. Since individuals are morally responsible for their conduct, deviant, and unpredictable behavior is bad conduct, and illness is the penalty for it.

Taboo Breaking

Yet another, related etiological category involves the breaking of a taboo:

> Theories which explain sickness as punishment sent by the gods for breach of religious prohibitions, or social prohibitions having divine sanction, fall under this heading. The breach may be quite unintentional, and even unknown, to the sufferer, but is nonetheless regarded as the real cause of his sickness (Clement, 1932, p. 188).

The attendant disorder(s) encompass a wide range of somatic and behavioral symptomatology: psychophysiological complaints such as mild weight loss, sleeplessness, fatigue, tissue edema, and headaches and heavy, irregular menstruation among women) and, on the other hand, marked mood variation, paranoia, and even epileptic-like seizures.

The precipitating breaches of taboo often seem to involve sexual behavior. Drawing upon Navajo mythology, Kaplan and Johnson (1964) sketch the course and outcomes of "moth sickness," *iich'aa,* which is said to be caused by brother-sister incest. Devereux (1939) reports a similar set of circumstances in Mohave communities. Hallowell (1939), continuing his emphasis upon illness as social sanction among the Ojibwa, relates fifteen case histories of mental disorders in which various forms of sexual aggression (autoerotism, homosexuality, certain aspects of heterosexuality, and bestiality) are posited as causal. Wallis and Wallis (1953) extend this explanation to the transgressors' descendents—at least among Canadian Dakota— arguing that they too may suffer. Eisenman (1965, 1967) essentially repeats Hallowell's conclusions in his review of Eskimo deviancy and taboo breaking. The literature is not limited to examples of sexual norm violation, but includes murder (Hallowell, 1936), deceit (Ritzenhaler, 1963), and neglected social obligations (Underhill, 1957) as well.

LaBarre (1947, 1964) attributes the resultant illness to personal guilt and fear. In classic psychodynamic fashion, he discusses it in terms of an admixture of superego anxiety with ego anxiety and the cathartic role of verbalization as confession.

Ghost Sickness

An etiological category not included within Clement's classification can be labeled generically as "ghost sickness," after the well-known Navajo disorder. Though related to the influence of evil power, it lacks the salient features peculiar to the other categories (spirit intrusion, soul loss, and breaking of taboo). Kaplan and Johnson (1964, p. 212) characterize the predominant symptoms as "weakness, bad dreams, feelings of danger, confusion, feelings of futility, loss of appetite, feelings of suffocation, fainting, dizziness, fear, and so forth." In a typical case,

the individual enters a period of anxiety and generalized fear. This fear seems to emanate from a feeling of helplessness and in some cases terror, which precedes and accompanies the involuntary eruption of unconscious impulses the individual has little or no control over his mind. He may have delusions about sights and sounds in the dark. He may have repetitive nightmares. He may have hallucinations. (Morgan, 1936, p. 7)

Wyman, Hill, and Osanai (1942, p. 377) and Johnson and Proskauer (1974) confirm this general pattern.

Fathauer (1951, p. 606) describes "ghost sickness" among the Mohave as a slight variant of *ghost-weyla.k*. The symptoms are as outlined above and derive from close physical proximity with the "the dead ones," usually portrayed as owls (see also Stewart, 1970). In a detailed set of papers on Apache reactions to and beliefs about death, Opler (1936, 1938, 1945, 1946) and Opler and Bittle (1961) recount a large number of cases within the Chiricahua, Mescalero, Jicarilla, Lipan, and Kiowa Apache communities that have similar manifestations and presumed etiology. Boyer (1964a, 1964b) corroborates Opler's observations and examines the psychodynamic implications that the *ch?idnoh*, "malevolent ghost," has for Apache personality development.

This brief review is, of course, far from exhaustive. The studies discussed herein provide some sense of the nature and diversity of conceptions of mental disorder among American Indians. However, for the most part, they represent an external view seldom informed by the sociocultural contexts in which such experiences are embedded as everyday life. Thus a given behavioral configuration may be misinterpreted in several different ways, leading to erroneous conclusions of pathology and dysfunction.

One kind of error follows from reliance upon a limited (and narrowly representative) set of informants. Consider, for example, Johnson and Johnson's (1965) treatment of *ta watl' yesni*. On the basis of interviews with two or three members of the Standing Rock Sioux Reservation, they interpreted it as "totally discouraged." A more complete inquiry shows that this utterance may also mean "tiredness" or "approaching with dread." *Ta watl' yesni* is an essentially descriptive phrase; one distinguishes felt intensity and pervasiveness from context.

Errors of this sort are often compounded by extension beyond the informant's experiential sphere to other, entire communities. For instance, *ta watl' yesni* has been used to describe similar behavioral configurations among the Cheyenne (Algonkian-speakers), Winnebago (a Siouan language group), and the Dakota-speaking Canadian Assiniboine. These tribes are linguistically distinct entities that may make wholly different psychosocial attributions to the *apparently* same set of behaviors.

Yet another error arises from failure to take the functional aspects of a phenomenon into account. The Lakota term *wacinko* is a case in point. It is now most commonly translated in reservation vernacular as "to pout." Lewis (1975), citing a wide range of symptoms including anger, withdrawal, psychomotor retardation, mutism, and immobility, concludes that wacinko constitutes a mild to severe reactive depressive illness. On the other hand, Siouan oral history and ethnographic observations—especially by native linguist Ella Deloria—indicate that the behavioral configuration in question is not necessarily a manifestation of pathology, but may serve practical ends:

> The Dakota managed to achieve privacy in their own adroit fashion. They made their own privacy, and it was mentally affected. . . . As for thinking one's thoughts in a crowded tipi, it was more possible to those accustomed to it than you might think. All tipi conversation was normally geared low for that purpose, with little excitement evident in the voice. The attitude of a speaker in group was generally not indicated so much by exclamatory outbursts and other generally not indicated so much by exclamatory outbursts and other variation of tone as by idiom. Thus anyone could withdraw from a group in spirit and think undisturbed, even with talking going on all about him. (Deloria, 1944 pp. 44, 46)

A number of examples of present-day transformations on wacinko as a form of individual autonomy in decision making are instructive:

(1) Babies throw theselves down upon the ground as an expression of willfulness. Observation of this behavior in infants six months onward have been noted.
(2) Children of either sex may wacinko to get away from troublesome siblings and overprotective parents.
(3) Teenagers may wacinko and move from a stressful home situation into the home of another member of the *tiospaye* (extended family).
(4) Males of all ages may wacinko to get away from wives and interact with male peers. (Currently, this often hereald the onset of a drinking spree.)
(5) Women may wacinko after a quarrel with a husband or lover who ultimately controls future interaction.

(6) Grandparents may wacinko if living in one child's home becomes too onerous and they wish to move to another's house.

There are many more examples of this "cultural-time-out" that are recognized and respected among the Lakota. Wacinko is used differentially and selectively. One need not ask, *"Ta ya un he(ho)?"* ("Is he/she in a state of well-being?" or, more correctly, "Is he/she competent?").

This last observation suggests an important point of departure for future research: cultural competence as defined and operationalized by native people. It encourages a focus on content, on indigenous theories of personhood, and ultimately, on successful psychosocial function as the interaction between both arenas. These seem to be the underlying dimensions of which instances of psychopathology afford only a partial understanding. Moreover, a reorientation of this nature shifts attention from improving inherently biased nosologies and psychological measures (Shore & Manson, in press) toward identifying the situations, developmental tasks, and skills required for an Indian person to meet particular needs and to achieve life goals in his or her own terms. Here, then, begins the search for alternative frameworks by which to conceptualize the relationship between American Indians and their mental health status. The search also should include efforts to discover prevention strategies that are consistent with Indian lifestyle orientations.

PREVENTIVE MENTAL HEALTH
IN INDIAN COMMUNITIES

Knowledge about preventive mental health among Indians has been handicapped by a lack of comparative research, particularly in the area of human competence (Manson, 1983). Even a cursory examination of the literature indicates that there has been little integration of psychological and anthropological theory and research on the subject of human competence (Dinges & Duffy, 1979; Dinges, Trimble, & Hollenbeck, 1979). It is interesting to speculate on the apparent reluctance to compare one culture with another in terms of relative effectiveness in producing competent persons. Perhaps this reluctance is based on the relativist posture of much of anthropological theory, which holds that cultures are doing their best at any given time to adapt to environmental demands. Berry (1975), for example, takes this position in his ecological approach to cross-cultural psychology by maintaining that no general criteria of cultural or behavioral excellence are possible.

The most influential theory of culture influence on mental health insofar as American Indians are concerned is that of Leighton (1961), who proposed a direct relationship between cultural disintegration and individual mental illness (compare Leighton & Leighton, 1941). In its simplest form, Leighton's theory holds that there is a universal striving for an "essential psychical condition" (EPC), which may be inhibited or facilitated by the culture.

The choice of factors indicative of cultural disintegration, which include migration, poverty, and "broken homes," all lead to generally negative predictions about the mental health of American Indians. By Leighton's standards it would be difficult to find many well-integrated Indian cultures, yet large-scale, broad-sample studies do not yield evidence for the epidemic proportion mental illness among these populations. Although systematic psychiatric epidemiological studies are only now becoming available, nationwide study of Indian youth indicates that

> they are not depressed, anxious, paranoid, or alienated as a group. They can make use of educational and economic opportunities. However, they do have the same problems other low-income groups have, and these problems are complicated to a degree by the fact that they are Indians. (Fuchs & Havighurst, 1972, p. 150)

The limitations of past psychopathology research become obvious when the goal of promoting competence among American Indians is considered. The basic problem appears to arise from the cul-de-sac into which traditional culture and psychopathology studies have led us. Perhaps one way out may be found in contemporary research areas that have been neglected, but may coincide more closely with indigenous theories of behavior. An illustration taken from the Navajo is instructive in this regard.

In his analysis of the nature of *nixch'i* "wind" concept as the central theoretical entity of the Navajo theory of life and behavior, McNeley (1975, p. 295-296) finds at least some basic aspects similar to current social learning theory:

> If the "wind within one" (nixch'i hwii'sizinii) as an immediate source of thought and behavior, be taken to refer in part to the same reality as an individual's repertoire of acquired or learned behaviors in social

learning theory, then both theories concur that this reality may be weakened or strengthened by means of external influences and experiences.

Although Navajo behavior theory and social learning theory would obviously differ at many levels, it is important to consider the implications for preventive mental health presented by a *rapprochement* between indigenous theories and those derived from entirely different epistomologies (for example, see Glidewell, 1972). Their potential convergence suggests a fruitful redirection of future research for purposes of promoting competence among American Indians.

SUMMARY

The perspectives taken in this chapter are consistent with growing challenges to the presumptive nature of many contemporary mental health practices. The anthropologist Hsu (1976, p. 157) typified the general mood when he asserted that "culture bound myopia has prevented our prominent social and clinical scientists from coming to grips with most other problems especially in the mental health fields."

Conventional Euro-American psychiatric and psychological mental health orientations need reform in terms of their relevance for Indian communities. Some practitioners argue for more studies that carefully examine the intrinsic nature of culture-specific syndromes (Bourguignon, 1979) and the role of traditional healers in delivering mental health services (Bergman, 1973; Dinges et al., 1981). Bourguignon (1979, p. 279) argues that the anthropologist, in particular, should attempt to "understand the societal control function of illness as well as the context of medical practice and belief."

Presumptions concerning etiology, diagnosis, and treatment of mental and behavioral disorders among American Indians must be reexamined in much greater depth and detail. The examination and analysis must recognize, first and foremost, the deeply entrenched way deviance is conceptualized in many Indian communities. A good beginning obviously is to conduct a small ethnography of values and beliefs and how they are tied into lifestyle patterns.

In our review of indigenous concepts of mental disorders we emphasized a multitude of classifications, symptom characteristics, and treatment forms. Perhaps the most important aspect of the review—one that demands strong emphasis—is the recognition that many of the indigenous concepts are undergoing changes in the way contemporary Indians view them. Many of the treatment styles, for example, are blends of some contemporary forms of counseling and psychotherapeutic approaches. Some healers, too, have been known to touch up their diagnoses with bits and pieces of psychodynamic theories. More important, many of the indigenous concepts are becoming more pan-Indian, accommodating perspectives from many different tribal groups. Therefore, it would behoove any non-Indian practitioner to understand the existing nature of indigenous diagnostic and treatment forms and not rely exclusively on past, historical depictions of mental disorders.

As researchers and practitioners seek to discover and reconceptualize perspectives toward indigenous concepts of mental health, intervention and prevention efforts will likely be affected. Institutional and organizational arrangements will also feel the pressure to change to accommodate new directions. Practitioners may find, for example, that the indigenous conceptualization and treatment of a disorder such as alcoholism may not be useful for treating addictive substances such as cocaine and heroin. In one Pacific Northwest Coast Salish community the "spirit healer" and the community alcohol treatment personnel have extreme difficulty generalizing their approaches to treating cocaine and marijuana—as a consequence the problem is ignored and goes untreated. The challenge for the practitioners in this community is to blend applicable elements of the existing traditional approach with adaptable drug treatment schemes. To accomplish this, though a number of small but significant changes may have to occur in the way yet another unfamiliar problem is dealt with in a traditional manner.

Finally, the biomedical tradition has dominated the field of mental health for too long. Continued efforts to comprehend mental and behavioral problems in many Indian areas from a biomedical approach will likely continue to be met with resistance. The resistance also translates into underutilization of services and antagonistic attitudes toward non-Indian mental health practitioners. Indigenous concepts of mental disorders must be examined for their intrinisic value and their linkage to culture-specific patterns of daily living. Theoretical and substantive advances can occur only if we explore the way modern approaches to mental health can accommodate the wisdom of indigenous approaches, creating a realistic blend that meshes with a traditional Indian world view.

REFERENCES

Aginsky, B. W. (1940). The socio-psychological significance of death among the Pomo Indians. *American Image, 1*(3), 1-11.

Attneave, C., & Kelso, D. (1977). *American Indian annotated bibliography of mental health* Volume 1. Seattle: Department of Psychology, University of Washington.

Balikci, A. (1963). Shamanistic behavior among the Ntsililk Eskimos. *Southwestern Journal of Anthropology, 19*, 380-396.

Barnouw, V. (1963). *Culture and personality.* Homewood, IL: Dorsey.

Bergman, R. L. (1973). Navajo medicine and psychoanalysis. *Human Behavior, 2* 8-15.

Berry, J. W. (1975). An ecological approach to cross-cultural psychology. *Nederlands Tijdschrift Voor De Psycholgie, 30*, 51-84.

Boag, T. A. (1970). Mental health of native peoples of the Arctic. *Canadian Psychiatric Association Journal, 15*, 115-120.

Bolman, W. M., & Katz, A. S. (1966). Hamburger hoarding: A case of symbolic cannibalism resembling whitiko psychosis. *Journal of Nervous and Mental Disorders, 142*, 424-428.

Bourguignon, E. (1979). *Psychological anthropology.* New York: Holt, Rinehart & Winston.

Boyer, L. B. (1964a). Folk psychiatry of the Apaches of the Mescalero Indian Reservation. In A. Kiev (Ed.), *Magic, faith and healing: Studies in primitive psychiatry today* (pp. 384-419). New York: Free Press.

Boyer, L. B. (1964b). Psychological problems of a group of Apaches: Alcoholic hallucinosis and latent homosexuality among typical men. *Psychoanalytic Study of Society, 3*, 203-277.

Brill, A. A. (1913) Piblokto or hysteria among Peary's Eskimos. *Journal of Nervous Mental Disorders, 40*, 514-520.

Brown, J. (1971). The cure and feeding of windigos: A critique. *American Anthropologist, 73*, 20-22.

Capron, L. (1953). The medicine bundles of the Florida Seminole and the Green Corn Dance (Anthropological Paper No. 35). *Bureau of American Ethology Bulletin, 151*, 159-210.

Clement, F. E. (1932). Primitive concepts of disease. *University of California Archaeology and Ethology, 32*, 185-252.

Cooper, J. M. (1932). Primitive concepts of disease. *University of California Archaeology and Ethology, 32*, 185-252.

Cooper, J. M. (1933). The Cree witiko psychosis. *Primitive Man, 6,* 20-24.

Dall, W. H. (1870). *Alaska and its resources.* Boston: Lee & Shepard.

Deloria, E. C. (1944). *Speaking of Indians.* New York: Friendship.

Devereux, G. (1937). Mohave soul concepts. *American Anthropologist, 39,* 417-422.

Devereux, G. (1939). The social and cultural implications of incest among the Mohave Indians. *Psychoanalytic Quarterly, 8,* 510-533.

Dinges, N., & Duffy, L. (1979). Culture and competence. In A. Marsella, R. Tharp, & T. Ciborowski (Eds.), *Perspectives in cross-cultural psychology* (pp. 209-232). New York: Academic.

Dinges, N., Trimble, J. E., & Hollenbeck, A. (1979). American Indian adolescent socialization: A review of the literature. *Journal of Adolescence, 2,* 259-296.

Dinges, N., Trimble, J., Manson, S., & Pasquale, F. (1981). The social ecology of counseling and psychotherapy with American Indians and Alaskan Natives. In A. Marsella & P. Pedersen (Eds.), *Cross-cultural counseling and psychotherapy: Foundations, evaluation, cultural considerations* (pp. 243-276). Elmsford, NY: Pergamon.

Eisenman, R. (1965). Scapegoating and social control. *Journal of Psychology, 61,* 203-209.

Eisenman, R. (1967). Scapegoating the deviant in two cultures. *International Journal of Psychology, 2*(2), 133-138.

Fathauer, G. H. (1951). The Mohave "ghost doctor." *American Anthropologist, 53,* 605-607.

Fogelson, R. (1965). Psychological theories of Windigo "psychosis," and a preliminary application of a model approach. In M. E. Spiro (Ed.), *Context and meaning in cultural anthropology* (pp. 74-99). New York: Free Press.

Foulks, E. F. (1973). The arctic hysterias of the North Alaskan Eskimo. *Abstracts International, 33* 2905B. (University Microfilms No. 73-1387, 425)

Freeman, D.M.A., Foulks, E. F., & Freeman, P. A. (1978). child development and Arctic hysteria in the North Alaskan Eskimo male. *Journal of Psychological Anthropology, 1,* 203-210.

Fuchs, E., & Havighurst, R. J. (1972). *To live on this earth: American Indian education.* Garden City, NY: Doubleday.

Furst, P. T. (1974). The roots and continuities of Shamanism. *Artscanada,* pp. 33-60.

Glidewell, J. C. (1972). A social psychology of mental health. In S. Golann & C. Eisdorfer (Eds.), *Handbook of community mental health* (pp. 211-248). New York: Appleton-Century-Crofts.

Gussow, Z. (1960). Pibloktoq (hysteria) among the Polar Eskimo: An ethno-psychiatric study. *Psychoanalytic Study of Society, 1,* 218-236.

Hallowell, A. I. (1934). Culture and mental disorder. *Journal of Abnormal and Social Psychology, 29*(1), 1-9.

Hallowell, A. I. (1936). Psychic stresses and culture patterns. *American Journal of Psychiatry, 92,* 1291-1310.

Hallowell, A. I. (1939). Sin, sex, and sickness in Saultaux belief. *British Journal of Medical Psychology, 18,* 191-197.

Hallowell, A. I. (1963). Ojibwa world view and disease. In I. Galdston (Ed.), *Man's image in medicine and anthropology.* New York: International Universities Press.

Hay, T. H. (1971). The windigo psychosis: Psychodynamic, cultural, and social factors in aberrant behavior. *American Anthropologist, 73*, 1-19.

Hsu, F.L.K. (1976). Rethinking our promises. In J. Westermeyer (Ed.), *Anthropology and mental health* (pp. 153-160). The Hague: Mouton.

Jenness, D. (1959). *The people of twilight.* Chicago: University of Chicago Press.

Jilek, W. G. (1974). Indian healing power: Indigenous therapeutic practices in the Pacific Northwest. *Psychiatric Annals, 4*(9), 13-21.

Jilek, W. G., & Jilek-Aall, L. (1971). A transcultural approach to psychotherapy with Canadian Indians: Experiences from the Fraser Valley of British Columbia. In *Psychiatry (Part II) Proceedings of the Fifth World Congress of Psychiatry* (pp. 1181-1186; Excerpta Medica International Congress Series, No. 274). Mexico City, Mexico.

Jilek, W. G., & Todd, N. (1974). Witchdoctors succeed where doctors fail: Psychotherapy among Coast Salish Indians. *Canadian Psychiatric Association Journal, 19*, 351-356.

Jilek-Aall, L. (1972). What is sasquatch—or, the problematics of reality testing. *Canadian Psychiatric Association Journal, 17*, 243-247.

Johnson, D. L., & Johnson, C. A. (1965). Totally discouraged: A depression syndrome of the Dakota Sioux. *Transcultural Psychiatric Research, 1*, 141-143.

Johnson, L. G., & Proskauer, S. (1974). Hysterical psychosis in a prepubescent Navajo girl. *Journal of the American Academy of Child Psychiatry, 13*, 1-19.

Jones, W. (1916). Ojibwa tales from the North Shore of Lake Superior. *Journal of American Folklore, 29.*

Kaplan, B., & Johnson, D. L. (1964). The social meaning of Navajo psychopathology and psychotherapy. In A. Kiev (Ed.), *Magic, faith and healing studies in primitive psychiatry today* (pp. 203-229). New York: Free Press.

Kiev, A. (1972). *Transcultural psychiatry.* New York: Free Press.

LaBarre, W. (1947). Primitive psychotherapy in Native American cultures: Peyotism and confession. *Journal of Abnormal and Social Psychology, 42*, 294-309.

LaBarre, W. (1964). Confession as cathartic therapy in American Indian tribes. In A. Kiev (Ed.), *Magic, faith and healing: Studies in primitive psychiatry today* (pp. 36-49). New York: Free Press.

Laidlaw, G. E. (1918). Ojibwa myths and tales, 30th Annual Archaeological Report, 1918. Appendix to *Report of the Minister of Education, Ontario* (pp. 74-110). Toronto: King's Printer.

Laidlaw, G. E. (1920). Ojibwa myths and tales, 32nd Annual Archaeological Report, 1920. Appendix to *Report of the Minister of Education, Ontario* (pp. 66-85). Toronto: King's Printer.

Laidlaw, G. E. (1927). Ojibwa myths and tales, 35th Annual Archaeological Report, 1924-25. Appendix to *Report of the Minister of Education, Ontario* (pp. 34-80). Toronto: King's Printer.

Landes, R. (1938a). The abnormal among the Ojibwa Indians. *Journal of Abnormal and Social Psychology, 33*, 14-33.

Landes, R. (1938b). *The Ojibwa women.* New York: Columbia University Press.

Leighton, A. H. (1961). Cultures as causative of mental disorder. In A. H. Leighton & H. J. Hughes (Eds.), *Causes of mental disorder: A review of epidemiological knowledge* (pp. 341-365). New York: Milbank Memorial Fund.

Leighton, A. H., & Leighton, D. C. (1941). Elements of psychotherapy in Navajo religion. *Psychiatry: Journal of the Biology and Pathology of Interpersonal Relations, 4*, 515-523.

Lewis, T. H. (1975). A syndrome of depression and mutism in the Ogalala Sioux. *American Journal of Psychiatry, 132*, 753-755.

Manson, S. M. (Ed.). (1983). *New directions in prevention among American Indian and Alaska native communities.* Portland: Oregon Health Sciences University.

Marano, L. (1982). Windigo psychosis: The anatomy of an emic/etic confusion. *Current Anthropology, 23*, 385-412.

McNeley, J. K. (1975). *The Navajo theory of life and behavior.* Unpublished doctoral dissertation, University of Hawaii.

Morgan, W. (1936). *Human wolves among the Navajo.* New Haven, CT: Yale University Press.

Murdock, G. P. (1965a). Tenino shamanism. *Ethnology, 4*, 165-171.

Murdock, G. P. (1965b). Tenino shamanism. *Transcultural Psychiatric Research, 2*, 144-146.

Nieuwenhuis, A. W. (1924). Principles of Indian medicine in American ethnology and their psychological significance. *Janus, 28*, 305-356.

Novakovsky, S. (1924). Arctic or Siberian hysteria as a reflex of the geographic environment. *Ecology, 5*, 113.

Opler, M. E. (1936). An interpretation of ambivalence of two American Indian tribes. *Journal of Social Psychology, 7*, 82-116.

Opler, M. E. (1938). Further comparative anthropological data bearing on the solution of a psychological problem. *Journal of Social Psychology, 9*, 477-483.

Opler, M. E. (1945). The Lipan Apache death complex and its extensions. *Southwestern Journal of Anthropology, 1*, 122-144.

Opler, M. E. (1946). Reaction to death among the Mescalero Apache. *Southwestern Journal of Anthropology, 2*, 454-467.

Opler, M. E., & Bittle, W. E. (1961). The death practices and eschatology of Kiowa Apache. *Southwestern Journal of Anthropology, 17*, 383-394.

Parker, S. (1960). The wittiko psychosis in the context of Ojibwa personality and culture. *American Anthropologist, 62*, 603-623.

Parker, S. (1962). Eskimo psychopathology in the context of Eskimo personality and culture. *American Anthropologist, 64*, 76-96.

Peary, R. E. (1910). *The North Pole.* New York: Frederick A. Stokes.

Rappaport, T. (1967). Ritual regulation of environmental relations among a New Guinea people. *Ethology, 16*, 17-30.

Ritzenthaler, R. (1945). The ceremonial destruction of sickness by the Wisconsin Chippewa. *American Anthropologist, 47*, 320-322.

Ritzenthaler, R. (1963). Primitive therapeutic practices among the Wisconsin Chippewa. In I. Galdston (Ed.), *Man's image in medicine and anthropology.* New York: International Universities Press.

Rohrl, V. J. (1970). A nutritional factor in windigo psychosis. *American Anthropologist, 72*, 97-101.

Saindon, J. E. (1933). Mental disorders among the James Bay Cree. *Primitive Man, 6*, 1-12.

Shore, J. H., & Manson, S. (in press). American Indian psychiatric and social problems. *Transcultural Psychiatric Research Review.*

Stewart, K. M. (1970). Mohave Indian shamanism. *Masterkey, 44,* 19-27.

Straight, W. M. (1970). Seminole Indian medicine. *Journal of the Florida Medical Association, 57*(8), 19-27.

Teicher, M. I. (1960). Windigo psychosis: A study of a relationship between belief and behavior among the Indians of Northeastern Canada. In V. F. Ray (Ed.), *Proceedings of the 1960 Annual Spring Meeting of the American Ethnological Society.* Seattle: University of Washington Press.

Trimble, J. E. (1981). Value differentials and their importance in counseling American Indians. In P. Pedersen, J. Draguns, W. Lonner, & J. Trimble, *Counseling across cultures.* Honolulu: University Press of Hawaii.

Trimble, J. E., & Medicine, B. (1976). Development of theoretical models and levels of interpretation in mental health. In J. Westermeyer (Ed.), *Anthropology and mental health* (pp. 161-200). The Hague: Mouton.

Underhill, R. (1957). Religion among American Indians. *Annals of the American Academy of Political and Social Science, 311,* 127-136.

Vallee, F. G. (1966). Eskimo theories of mental illness in the Hudson Bay region. *Anthropologica, 8,* 53-83.

Wallace, A.F.C. (1961). Mental illness, biology and culture. In F.L.K. Hsu (Ed.), *Psychological anthropology: Approaches to culture and personality* (pp. 225-295). Homewood, IL: Dorsey.

Wallace, A.F.C., & Ackerman, R. E. (1960). An interdisciplinary approach to mental disorder among the polar Eskimos of northwest Greenland. *Anthropologica, 2*(1).

Wallis, R. S., & Wallis, W. D. (1953). The sins of the fathers: Concept of disease among the Canadian Dakota. *Southwestern Journal of Anthropology, 9,* 431-435.

Weyer, E. M. (1932). *The Eskimos.* New Haven, CT: Yale University Press.

Whiting, B. B. (1950). *Piaute sorcery.* New York: Viking Fund.

Whitney, H. (1911). *Hunting with the Eskimos.* New York: Century.

Wyman, L., Hill, W. W., & Osanai, M. (1942). Navaho eschatology. *University of New Mexico Bulletin, 377.*

9

MENTAL HEALTH SERVICE DEVELOPMENT
The Case of Indonesia

THOMAS W. MARETZKI

The purpose of this chapter is to raise questions about the relationship of basic research in culture and mental health to the needs for information and decisions related to policies and service delivery in the national mental health system of a non-Western country, Indonesia. Raising questions might offer food for thought to researchers. My position is that there has been little feedback from the findings and ideas that have been generated by social scientists to confront the challenges of mental health service development in which culture plays a central part.

The explanation for this state of affairs can be found in several factors. The basis for mental health service planning is determined by existing needs, by available and proven experiences elsewhere within a system of internationally recognized standards of practice, and by proven approaches to the most urgent problems of psychiatric care. Until recently, none of these could be found in traditional cultural studies by anthropologists, in part because none of the cultural studies addressed situations faced by practical mental health planners. A reason for this is the totally separate spheres in which research of this kind takes place and is disseminated. It is outside the range of information available and relevant to planning, policymaking, and service delivery for the health sector. This situation could change as new conceptual approaches and methods are developed in the social and behavioral sciences linking research to an awareness of clinical situations and appropriate methodologies, as well as to an awareness of the reality of medical systems (in a broad cultural sense and including the modern cosmopolitan medical system). These changes, as they coincide with modified orientations toward a primary health care focus, open a potential for merging interests.

That mental health services should involve cultural considerations is not disputed in Indonesia (Setyonegoro, 1964; Salan & Maretzki, in press). In what way leadership or responsibility should be assumed, and who should assume it, may be less clear (Sampoerno, 1980). In a formal administrative sense the responsibility lies with the Director of Mental Health in the Ministry of Health. In that position Indonesia, at present, has a leader with a broad perspective on mental health. That Western-style services are in some instances inappropriate, unaffordable, far beyond the horizons of social and cultural—as well as economic—reality and existing human resources, and are potentially disruptive, as has been claimed (Higginbotham, 1979), is at best an oversimplication of many complex factors, most of which cannot be argued in this short discussion. The fact is that a basic health care and health service structure, which includes mental health services, is administratively established in Indonesia, a relatively recently independent and technologically developing country. There are still a number of options, which, it would seem, have long been lost in high-technology countries, where overspecialization and professionalism account for the kinds of services that are provided. While the Western model is not appropriate, reconciling innovative strategies with realities presents many puzzles. The recognition of viable and culturally appropriate options is itself a cultural matter that rests with Indonesians rather than outsiders.

The transfer of a Western medical model into a non-Western country is a historical fact that Indonesia shares with most other countries in Asia. In briefly reviewing the development of some ideas and practices in the emerging mental health services of a newly independent country, my presentation draws on the very limited knowledge of an outsider. Given certain facts—such as the administrative structures of health and mental health planning and present services, national goals and economic capacities, international organizations such as the World Health Organization (WHO), as well as professional considerations—on the one hand, and the useful knowledge and research results available, as well as attitudes that influence utilization of knowledge on the other, how can decision makers choose the best option?

Foster (1977) reviewed some of the phases of international aid as they relate to transition from the cultural imperialism of the Western donors in health fields. Beginning with a direct transfer of the medical technological system of donor nations, the medical model of the West was followed by a public health model that considered social, cultural, and psychological characteristics of the recipients. To this was recently added a general and formal recognition of cultural, social, and psychological factors inherent in the organizations involved in innovations. It has been suggested that the culture of bureaucracies can create barriers against the development of culture-appropriate services, independent of resistances at the levels of communities.

The emergence of philosophies in different parts of the Indonesian health system is beyond the scope of this presentation, but it is clear that a public and community health approach is the basis for the current national health system as reflected in the third Indonesian Five-Year Plan. Predating the 1978 WHO Alma Ata declaration, but greatly boosted by it, this approach is very responsive in principle to input from the community. The orientation of a Western-influenced curative medical system that has to provide basic technical services in a health system and the quite different orientation of a community public health approach that is more attuned to cultural variations naturally present enormous challenges when the two are merged. This must be recognized in the case of Indonesian mental health services developments, which are basically rooted in a psychiatric service model.

The psychiatrically based mental health system, responsive as it is to cultural input and recently to community health approaches through community psychiatry, now faces a great challenge in establishing connections with other systems. The system must provide the appropriate linkages from family and community-based health behaviors and related cultural systems to the established network of modern health facilities, of which the most basic is the community health clinic *(puskesmas)*. With community mental health as a bridge, there is at present a fluid situation for the established mental health system. This is reflected in a general openness to any useful and practical input to the existing system that can aid the improvement of mental health services. Here is one situation with which meaningful culture and mental health research could begin to articulate.

There are other significant contextual issues emanating from various social science orientations, which I can only mention briefly.

Critics of some of the excesses of psychiatry as the medical specialty assuming dominance in the curing of mental illness in Western countries have stirred responsive cords among some anthropologists who are familiar with different cultures and their management of divergent behaviors and emotional states. My approach, which accepts historical facts and the realities of the contemporary distribution of service responsibilities, may seem to such critics to be a captured point of view. My position is this: When there was a need to deal with the demands for immediate mental health services, what specialties were ready and able to initiate practical, effective, humane services, except for psychiatry? This position does not rule out a shift from the existing model to alternatives in which psychiatry will play a continued important role.

The development of the present mental health system in Indonesia took place during the last three decades, initially following the custodial care services of the preceding colonial administration. This recent period coincides with productive research growth in culture and mental health as a subfield of anthropology and transcultural psychiatry (Marsella, 1979; Maretzki, 1979). Neither the orientation of most researchers nor the nature of their findings meshed with the ongoing mental health services development in Indonesia or other countries. Anthropologists were still theoretically involved with methodologies appropriate to establish ethnic and cross-cultural validity. The concern was not with the nature and clinical considerations of mental health services.

The gap between basic and applied research is evident in culture and mental health. Most work is conducted as basic research. For example, we can consider the impact on psychiatry and mental health services of the federally funded culture and mental health research exchange program at the East-West Center and University of Hawaii between 1964 and 1972. In my opinion, there was little potential feedback of practical value. The main benefit lay in an exchange of experiences and the concentration on topics such as a review of indigenous therapy approaches in the final conference (Lebra, 1976). The program and conferences may have generated considerable sensitivity toward their own cultures among indigenous psychiatrists trained in the West, or a reinforcement of existing cultural values in relation to their psychiatric practice (Lapuz, 1973). This was the time when serious reevaluation of Western cultural dominance abounded.

Taking some other products of culture- and mental health-related research of the last two decades, where could planners and policy-makers have looked for stimulation and ideas to be translated into the needs of a culturally pluralistic nation? A very basic issue is the distinction between the classifications of diseases, in particular mental diseases, according to a standardized, worldwide applicable classification system (needed for statistical comparisons and general planning baselines), and the indigenous conception of disorders with which it never overlaps (Murphy & Leighton, 1965). This dilemma is widely recognized and efforts toward culturally sensitive and valid epidemiologies have been attempted (Carstairs & Kapur, 1976). Closely related is the area of culturally diverse thresholds and recognition of mental illness (Edgerton, 1969). More recently, the research of Katz and his associates has illustrated the relative perception of deviance according to diverse cultural orientations toward behavioral thresholds that separate normal from abnormal, and how this recognition translates into mental health services of a multicultural community (Katz, Sanborn, Lowerey, & Ching, 1978). Another example is seen in the responses of mental illness in different cultural contexts as explained by the role of labeling in differential recovery as an outcome (Waxler, 1977). Even more closely linked to clinical considerations are the results of research on the semantics of illness phenomena (Good, 1977; Good & Good, 1981). They suggest the significance of culturally sensitive response systems in health care. Finally, there is recognition of quite diverse culturally founded overall conceptions of mental health that shape entire treatment systems and approaches (Townsend, 1978). It is also clear that the distinction of mental health from health is arbitrary if viewed from a cross-cultural perspective since it does not exist as a differentiation in non-Western medical belief categories and behaviors.

Together with medical sociologists, some anthropologists have reflected on limitations imposed on their research by working from within medical institutions. Medical and administrative health settings for research offer insights parallel to those anthropologists claim as participant observers in any other cultural setting. Much as medical researchers such as Fabrega have carried clinical sensitivities into cultural settings, anthropologists bring cultural sensitivities into clinical environments. The studies of Caudill (1958), Fox (1959), and Gaines (1979) are examples. Kleinman's (1980) clinically oriented, ethnomedically based study of patients and healers is a successful model since it points the way to practical outcome and follow-up approaches. In Indonesia, studies of the cultural significance of mental health services would be useful. They would require a combination of anthropological methodology and conceptualization and clinically sensitive and relevant approaches.

Kleinman (1978) has argued in several papers the practical implications of ethnomedical research for international health planning. Others address ethnomedical and cultural illness perspectives in related ways. I summarize here four relevant theoretical notions of the ethnomedical model that provide directions for future research strategies:

(1) the disease/illness dichotomy that delimits specific illness problems and suggests interventions to prevent and manage them (Kleinman, 1978);

(2) the analysis of universal and culture-specific therapeutic relationships in terms of social constructions and negotiations of "clinical realities" and other clinical components and functions (Marsella & Pedersen, 1981);

(3) the concept of semantic illness networks and its relationship to health-seeking behavior (Good, 1977);

(4) the analysis of therapeutic efficacy as entailing inherent lay and practitioner conflicts in evaluating the "curing" of disease and "healing" of illness (Kleinman, 1980).

THE INDONESIAN CASE

I shall outline key factors in explaining the development of Indonesian mental health services by citing some facts, abstracting some important events, and relating some culturally relevant factors to what could have been considered in the past, or what might be considered in the future, as linking community needs and health policies and services.

With a population of nearly 150 million people, Indonesia, consisting of large and small islands, is stretched over a length of about 3400 miles and a width of about 1000 miles, the world's most extensive archipelago under one flag. There are an estimated 250 different languages spoken. Although some ethnic groups account for large proportions of the Indonesian population, for example, Javanese (about 50 percent), Sudanese (about 15 percent), Minangkabau,

Batak, Balinese, and others are centrally represented in government, education, and other national affairs. With many other groups of different cultural traditions, and also Chinese and Eurasians, there is no one Indonesian cultural solution. However, Indonesian as a national language and an Indonesian national identity emerge gradually; urbanization and rapid culture change in various areas of the country exposes different groups to comparable experiences.

While the dominant religion is Moslem, the degree of orthodoxy varies. There are Indonesian Christians in all parts of the country. Bali's population is mostly Hindu, but there are also Chinese who are Buddhist. Local traditional belief systems and religious orientations remain important aspects of life. The Ministry of Religion, with the largest staff of all Indonesian ministries, has the national task of regulating the roles and relationships of the diversity of religious streams.

Indonesia gained independence in 1945. In 1965, a major revolution established new government leadership. Through elections and representative legislative bodies the present government has gradually expanded democratic processes according to Indonesian principles. The governors and provincial governments collaborate closely with the central administration and rely on a central planning process that has an impact on the entire country. At present, Indonesia is in its third Five-Year Development Plan. The plan for mental health specifies the integration of services at the health centers and general hospitals, the reorganization of mental health service units, and the proper utilization of mental health workers. Centralization and the Five-Year Plan as a guiding instrument allow for the delivery of health services in each province to reflect local differences and requirements. The participation of communities is acknowledged as necessary for achieving mental health goals. However, the reality for mental health services is that, as part of the national health services, the responsibility is vested in administrators who have medical and/ or public health qualifications.

In Indonesia no one traditional medical system prevailed in any of the cultural areas prior to Western influence. Principles of Aryuvedic medicine, which were brought by travelers and traders from India, left a strong cultural mark on parts of Indonesia. They are reflected today in Javanese and Balinese traditional health beliefs and practices. In both areas these traditions are set down in books and manuals *(usada)* that focus on the art of healing (Koentjaraningrat, 1979; Goris, 1957). The usada, written in Kavi on bamboo rolls, are to this day consulted as the basis for action by the Balinese healers *(balian)* and the Javanese healer *(dukun)* (Leimena and Thong, 1979; Thong, 1980; Dipojono, 1979b; Suparlan, 1978; Hirokoshi-Roe, 1979). Unani medical principles are integrated with Moslem folk and religious practices as these are transmitted by religious teachers and leaders. Chinese medical knowledge is not only used by Chinese specialists, but has spread into other sectors, for example, in the practice of acupuncture in the folk sector as well as in the cosmopolitan medical centers.

The role of Javanese mysticism as reflected in the medically related activities of spiritual groups *(kebatinan),* is another major factor in Javanese culture and of significance in the area of mental health (Dipojono, 1972; 1979a, 1979b). The influence of a single major tradition, or of their combinations, further mixed with influences from a more basic Javanese folk tradition *(abangan)* is complex and changing (Geertz, 1960). Similar complexities apply to other, geographically more distant areas that have been less studied and are therefore less well known for contemporary health beliefs and practices. The situation is extremely varied and will require years of systematic study.

Local traditional folk healers and popular healers are widespread and function as an alternative health care base for the majority of Indonesians, including those who are well educated. New types of healers emerge in an ever-changing kaleidoscope of cultural mixes occurring through contacts and innovations. As these healers provide health and mental health care for such large numbers of Indonesians today, regardless of local background and education, they absorb new knowledge and practices—for example, from the cosmopolitan medical system—and integrate some of these into their practices (Salan & Maretzki, in press). In the attempt to capture this complexity there is a difficulty in separating genuine traditions that have been handed down from generation to generation (Subroto, 1979) from new and popular modifications.

Traditional cultural healing is carried out by specialists in the major cultural areas, Java, Sunda, Bali, and some in Sumatra, who can be subdivided into different categories according to the major principles of their specialized activities (Subroto, 1979; Dipojono, 1979a, 1979b; Suparlan, 1978; Leimena and Thong, 1979). A general categorization of healers distinguishes between those who practice as traditional midwives, as bone setters and massage experts, as herbalists, as predictors of the future or as numerologists, as practitioners of magic, and as practitioners who gain and utilize their knowledge on the basis of shamanistic practices. While these specializations can be conceptually separated, they often coexist, in part, in one individual practitioner. Clients look for a set of different individual diagnoses and their formulations, and incidentally for the specific cures that go with each. This explains much of the continued seeking of advice from a variety of traditional healers (Kalangie, 1980).

Western or cosmopolitan medicine appears as the most recently imported major medical system in Indonesia. Introduced by the Dutch colonial administration, it provided the mental health sector with custodial institutional care for the most severe cases of mental disorders, much as in other parts of the world where Western government style was superimposed on existing systems. This colonial system of mental health institutions was the legacy for the newly independent Indonesian government. It is a major factor in the realities and constraints of some of the events as they have taken shape and continue to develop in mental health.

The basic responsibility for the maintenance of government mental health services is vested in medical professionals. The combination of psychiatry as a medical specialization and a hospital-based services system has given mental health services the character they have today. On the basis of historical facts, especially the rise of science as a dominant, separate field of knowledge, it is difficult to imagine how modern mental health services could have been initially developed in such a way that psychiatry was *not* the dominant professional specialty. The most obvious and urgent problems were severe disorders, many with organic components. It is reasonable to ask (and the answer would depend on one's view of the ability and readiness of other specializations), where but in medical care could the responsibility and response readiness needed for serious mental disturbances be placed?

In Indonesia this question has never been raised seriously until the present (Sampoerno, 1980). The problem is tied to the basic conceptualization of mental health and mental illness in relation to health and illness in general. Given the hindsight of historical developments, and new insights and explorations of alternatives, a conceptual distinction between the role of the clinical medical sciences and public health has emerged. It seeks at all levels, especially in mental health, a workable linkage approach. Within psychiatry, the absorption in the West and diffusion to other parts of the world of more social and culturally oriented perspectives has provided a basis for internal shifts. These are evident in Indonesia. If we look at the present realities of mental health services developments in Indonesia, the efficiency of the developing system must be judged in terms of potential alternatives in order to make the consideration of future complimentary approaches possible.

The basis for mental health services in Indonesia today is contained in a basic mental health law (Undang undang Tentang Kesehatan Jiwa 1966/No. 9), which, in turn, has its roots in basic health legislation. The original structure of the government mental health system has remained relatively unchanged, since the Directorate of Mental Health is part of the Directorate General for Medical Care in the Ministry (see Figure 9.1).

A nation-wide hospital-based system has under present leadership been developed into a strong, responsive, and unfolding system of mental health services that begins to build links into the government-established community health centers (*puskesmas*) (Setyonegoro, 1980). The government system in 1981 offered 7000 beds in 24 provincial hospitals and was bolstered by an additional bed capacity of university hospitals and a rapidly increasing average of 10 psychiatric beds targeted for each of about 250 general hospitals throughout the country by 1982.

The staffing and care of the government mental hospital and general hospital facilities (including outpatient facilites in both), and increasingly those in selected community health centers, rest primarily with the psychiatric and other professional staff of the Directorate of Mental Health. While this system need not be described here, it's unusual feature is the fact that, unlike in all other health care services in Indonesia, the mental health staff of the public sector reports to the director of mental health in the Ministry of Health. Therefore, it can respond directly to a centralized approach while retaining simultaneously a close working relationship with the local, provincial, and lower-level health sectors throughout the country.

This system has been recognized as unusual for a developing country in a number of ways. An example is the existence of a national computerized mental health registry system that records all cases diagnosed and treated within the system that are part of the Directorate (that is, the mental hospitals). Other examples are the

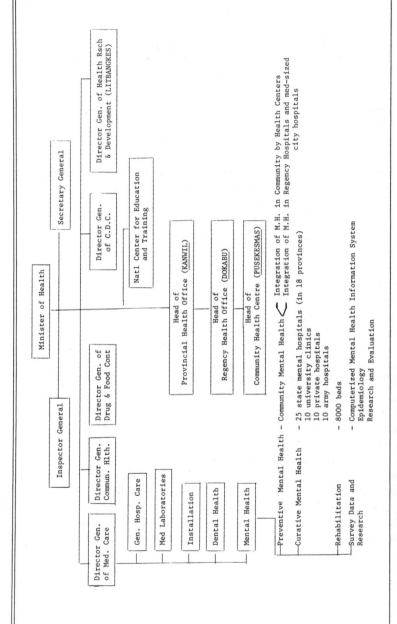

Figure 9.1 The Structure of the Indonesian Health Department

Minister of Health

Inspector General

Secretary General

Director Gen. of Med. Care

Director Gen. Commun. Hlth.

Director Gen. of Drug & Food Cont

Director Gen. of C.D.C.

Director Gen. of Health Rsch & Development (LITBANGKES)

Natl Center for Education and Training

Head of Provincial Health Office (KANWIL)

Head of Regency Health Office (DOKABU)

Head of Community Health Centre (PUSEKESMAS)

Gen. Hosp. Care

Med Laboratories

Installation

Dental Health

Mental Health

Preventive Mental Health – Community Mental Health — Integration of M.H. in Community by Health Centers

Integration of M.H. in Regency Hospitals and med-sized city hospitals

Curative Mental Health — 25 state mental hospitals (in 18 provinces)
10 university clinics
10 private hospitals
10 army hospitals

— 8000 beds

Rehabilitation

Survey Data and Research — Computerized Mental Health Information System
Epidemiology
Research and Evaluation

231

responses to such unfolding needs as the use of appropriate medication, the treatment of drug abuse, child mental health, and, most importantly, for our discussion community psychiatry. All of these are coordinated centrally, but can amply respond to regional and local needs. In this unique adminstrative structure—where mental health chiefs in the different provinces are directly responsible to the director rather than to each provincial health chief—innovative leadership is at an advantage. It permits esprit de corps, a joint approach to problem solving, unified channels for communications and new ideas, and opportunities for coordinated efforts to help other sectors in the government or the private sector deal with mental health-related needs. This is demonstrated by the recently established Community Mental Health Development Board in the special province of Jakarta, which may be replicated in other provinces (Martono & Heerjan, 1980; Martono, Heerjan, & Harahap, 1980).

The close links between government psychiatric services and medical education in Indonesia began under a Dutch rule with heavy biological and neurological emphases. The cultural elements of psychiatric phenomena attracted Europe-an specialists since Kraeplin (1904). Among the Dutch, van Wulfften-Palthe (1948), a psychiatrist and head of the psychiatric service in Java, developed a research-oriented approach to the psychiatric conditions encountered in which other researchers from Europe became interested. Of these, Wolfgang Pfeiffer (1971) of Germany was the most culturally oriented during the more recent period. None of these had a direct and lasting impact on the development of Indonesia's developing medical education, although Pfeiffer's research contributed much to transcultural psychiatry in general. Meanwhile, Indonesian psychiatrists developed their own culturally oriented research, which they published in the national psychiatric journal, *Jiwa.*

A psychiatric specialization has developed in Indonesia during the last twenty years. There are now about 150 trained physicians in psychiatry, many with three years (some four) of psychiatric residency training completed. For some, their specialty training included extensive neurology training, but neurology is diminishing as part of psychiatric training in more recent postgraduate education.

The link with government mental health services is provided in two ways: All physicians, following graduation from medical school, are required to provide government services, and many of them are recruited into psychiatry as a specialization. Following or, for some, concurrent with their training, they work in government services as mental health specialists. The collaboration between medical faculties in psychiatry who are government employees (Ministry of Higher Education) and the psychiatrists in the mental health service (Ministry of Health) is so close that in many centers their activities overlap, since specialty clinical training is often based in government mental health hospitals. As a result, there are practically no sharp divisions between medical faculties in psychiatry and government psychiatrists. All participate in a unified objective and individuals move, to some extent, between the two systems even though in terms of appointments there are clear distinctions. The flow of ideas in psychiatry from the academic sector to those in the government sector is smooth and there are frequent contacts for stimulation and feedback into the academic setting. Indonesian medical education has developed in the interest of appropriate national health care.

How Western ideas initially influenced the academic (including psychiatric) professions, can be gauged from the writings of the former dean of the faculty of psychiatry at the University of Indonesia (a psychiatrist), where therapy approaches were originally developed. He regretted what he called the "materialistic organic point of view" to which physicians tenaciously adhered; he saw physicians as being refractory to accepting the importance of mental health influences (Santoso, 1959), and pointed out the need to introduce modern (Western) psychotherapy into Indonesia practice. As a further example of how much Western thinking at this point influenced educators, the same writer speculated that Javanese are relatively free of neuroses. It is therefore clear that the significant ideas with regard to the role of Indonesian cultural principles in Indonesia, some of which have been outlined by Dipojono (1979a, 1979b) are influenced by notions of a Western-educated and -oriented elite that tends to substitute foreign ideas for significant cultural heritage. Indonesian psychiatrists, like so many other educated persons in Indonesia and in other non-Western countries, live simultaneously in two cultural settings that are difficult to reconcile: their own as Indonesians of various ethnic affiliations, and their professional identity, which is quite obviously shaped by the requirements of the modern medical profession based on a Western model.

Community psychiatry, and how it relates to more general considerations, is a special focus for this discussion. It demonstrates

most clearly the conscious Indonesian emphasis of Indonesian
solutions to Indonesian problems. This gain in a separate identity and
independent grasp of situations and problems is an emergent characteristic of national significance. For community psychiatry the
crucial factor is the broader context of community-oriented health
care, which has become national policy. The emphasis of the national
Indonesian health system, and of basic medical education throughout Indonesia, has shifted to a community health- and public
health-oriented approach. Primary health care, here meaning health
care appropriate to the individual community level (not just the
development of certain medical specialization as they contribute to
needed health care as in the West), is the emphasis for this developing
country. Culture potentially plays a central part since existing beliefs
and practices in the community are a basic element in developing
needed and desired health care. The role of traditional healing is
clearly recognized. In the words of the director of mental health:

> It is exactly this cultural dimension which many health professionals in
> the past tended to overlook that now emerges as a major area of
> concern.

> In the field of mental health, in other words, it is therefore not only a
> matter of overt or formal psychopathology of mental or emotional
> disorder, or the question of culture bound syndromes, or the frequency
> of mental disorders that are important. It might be quite possible for a
> delivery system of community mental health care that these so-called
> "exotic phenomena", too, have practical implications. Viewed from
> this angle, we feel that both public health as well as mental health, may
> very well benefit from such approaches. (Directorate of Mental
> Health, 1979)

To this point in time, leadership in exploring the cultural and
related aspects of community psychiatry, and more generally
national mental health in all its implications, has rested with the
Directorate of Mental Health, and with medical faculties in psychiatry.
Conceivably, it will be vigorously explored and translated into
programs and actions, teaching, research planning and the like in
different parts of the Ministry of Health (such as the Institute of
Health Research and Development) and in faculties (such as public
health, anthropology, sociology, and others). My examples are
drawn from the recent effort in the Directorate of Mental Health.

Two recent national conferences are examples of a broad exploration of ideas suitable for actions to translate mental health services into culturally relevant and appropriate community-based mental health (and general health) care. Each gathering by invitation from the Directorate of Mental Health brought together provincial health chiefs and some of their staff with provincial mental hospital directors, specialists from faculties of medicinal schools and of public health, and from the social sciences in the main university centers thoughout the country. Also invited were other Ministry of Health administrators and key persons from other sectors of government. A few foreign consultants and anthropologists were invited to explore with the participants their knowledge of contemporary approaches and views, and the significance for recognition of cultural principles in health care delivery. From the perspective of academic social science in the West, it was a unique experience to find out that a group of over 200 practitioners and academicians, twice within a period of 18 months, were able to consider theories and findings in relations to what they laid out as the existing situation. A key to these conferences were the original research contributions and reports of Indonesian açademicians and practitioners in the health fields that assessed conditions and needs for additional knowledge (Directorate of Mental Health, 1978, 1979).

If there is contained in these explorations one overriding issue, it is the link between existing mental health services as they reach into the community health centers, and individual, family, and community conceptualizations of behaviors, emotions, states of well-being or stress, and deviancy, as these are translated into behavioral actions and help seeking. Given the size of the Indonesian population and worldwide mental illness statistics, as many as 1.5 million persons may be in need of direct psychiatric services for serious disturbances by Western diagnostic criteria and standards. The number of others who feel a need or demonstrate a need for help in what can be viewed as belonging to the broad realm of mental health is open-ended, and with it the nature of needed preventive and interventive mental health support. Assuming that the earlier tasks in developing responses to mental health needs lay in the control of severe disorders, and asserting that some of this control has been achieved in part with the help of psychoactive drugs and a variety of concomitant, although variably effective therapeutic approaches, the new frontier clearly lies at the community-service level. It is at this particular point that we may return to the question of what useful knowledge and experiences can be extracted or projected from the past and ongoing research efforts in culture and mental health.

An example for the anthropological role in linking health policies and social-cultural expertise is contained in the statement by the minister of health in opening the conference on traditional healing. He stressed the key role of the basic community structure, which he referred to as the *banjar* (the smallest social unit above the family in Balinese community structure), because it was in Bali that this unit proved to be an effective vehicle for a community-based approach to family planning. For anthropologists, this raises concerns about potential generalizations of experiences from one cultural community to others (Colfer, 1979). The question of the true locus of community-based health care is of central importance (Iskandar & Rienks, 1981).

The traditional folk and popular healing sectors are the major cultural stage where health beliefs and practices are in evidence. While they are accessible to the kind of objective information gathering needed at this stage, the other cultural stage, the family, is less so. Both have been the subjects of research by Indonesians and foreigners in Indonesia (Kalangie, 1980; McCauley, 1979; Connor, 1982; Directorate of Mental Health, 1978, 1979; Thong, 1980; Salan & Maretzki, in press). A future strategy for research should provide basic cultural information that could be translated into epidemiological baseline data, health education, community communications, and other practical approaches for mental health care.

I suggest, after personal observation in Indonesia, together with Indonesian psychiatrists and foreign psychiatrists, of diagnostic and curing practices by traditional healers that unless such research is carried out in conjunction with medical specialists, it is difficult to establish the necessary linkages among traditional diagnostic categories, corresponding healing, and the Western conceptualization of problems and modern alternative approaches.

A brief (not systematic or research-based) observation of a traditional healer treating a young woman provides the following example: The patient, brought to the healer by her family, had within the previous week experienced a sudden but drastic mood and behavior change. She was distraught, refused to engage in talk with her family, had considerably reduced food intake, slept irregularly, and in various other ways communicated to her family and to others, including the healer, severe distress. Treatment in a community health center without a mental health component proved unsatisfactory (apparently it merely consisted of an injection of vitamin B-12). The healer gave a diagnosis of bewitchment and suggested treatment at his house (along with other clients) for about two weeks.

While this case was not followed, as in systematic research it should be, and no formal psychiatric diagnosis was attempted, the discussion of the observers following a brief observation of the patient centered around possible differential psychiatric diagnoses and appropriate related intervention. It is at this level—in dealing with such phenomena, which are widespread in Indonesia—that systematic knowledge may help to identify more accurately what is appropriately handled in the existing folk sector, and what might alternatively or more appropriately be handled in the formal health care sector. Such research goes beyond the narrower confines of traditional culture and mental health research.

Related to these questions are those raised again and again with respect to phenomena in Indonesia about the role of altered states of consciousness in ordinary behavior of individuals, as well as in behaviors that have psychiatric connotations (Thong, 1980; Pfeiffer, 1971; Maretzki, 1981).

FUTURE DIRECTIONS

The transfer of a medical specialty originating in Western cultures to deal with mental health problems in Indonesia creates a set of complex realities for planners and practitioners. I have outlined some key factors that may help us view the Indonesian case against knowledge available through the social sciences and cross-cultural orientations in psychiatry, and the realities of the emerging situation.

Among reality factors, I have cited cultural diversity of the national population, no dominant traditional medical system, a legacy of a mental health system initially oriented toward acute and chronic patients with severe disorders, and changes arising from the beginning of an independent nation. Within two decades, the example of a narrowly focused Western conceptualized system of mental health intervention has yielded to a broader community mental health approach and an orientation toward primary care in which individual communities will play a strong part. This situation can now be linked to the changing knowledge base in the social sciences, particularly psychological and medical anthropology.

The dilemma for the Indonesian mental health services is that even if the core of seriously disturbed individuals is reached, how far do the responsibilities of the modern mental health system extend? How far should they extend in responding to broader needs when there is a limitation to available human resources and apparently an adaptive utilization of non-Western folk medical and other religious alternatives? This must be considered against the background of social and cultural changes affecting not only the urban centers, but also rural areas throughout most of the nation. Such challenges lead to a search for existing knowledge that could be applied in this situation, and an exploration of the potential role of traditional healers to provide linkages. Indonesia does not have a systematically developed culture-based mental health model that it can adapt generally, although Bali may be coming close. Mental health and other health officials seek culture-based practical research findings to generate adaptive strategies that will lead to solutions that are not harmful to clients or perhaps (and this is an unresolved issue) to limitation or control of traditional healers. What can Indonesia gain from the experiences elsewhere in the world and the accumulated knowledge based on these experiences?

The development of basic concepts and theoretical formulations that can be translated into behavioral dimensions of healthy individuals, identified clients or patients, and healers or health professions is essential for communications between researchers and practitioners and for potential feedback. Examples of some useful concepts are as follows: health care system, the distinction of disease and illness, labeling, health-seeking behavior, and semantic network. All of these have been used in clinically relevant ethnomedical research. Any of these concepts can be related to situations faced by people in need of responses to health/mental health problems, and apply equally to practitioners who are consulted, family members, traditional and popular healers, and modern health care professionals.

Examples of other basic research that could be of practical value are studies of concepts and dimensions of emotions, concepts of functioning and malfunctioning behavior and personality qualities, and the interactions of patients and practitioners (see Marsella, 1979, 1980; Marsella & Pedersen, 1981).

Finally, I have pointed to the importance of the culture of administrative systems in the innovative acceptance of, or the nature of political influences on, new ideas and approaches. Here options are, indeed, a part of the Indonesian reality. Professional specializations have not yet developed to the point where all considerations are influenced or determined by professional and economic niches as they are in the established West. Important as they may seem in respect to human rights, insurance considerations and legalistic complexities are not yet the basis for decisions that determine the course of mental health strategies in Indonesia.

Dr. Kusumanto Setyonegoro, the director of mental health, in his discussion of cultural distinctions between Western and non-Western cultures, emphasizes the analytical approaches of academic medicine that contrast with the holistic orientation of traditional healing systems. We are well aware of this issue as a focus for medical anthropology research. This may continue to be a key area of challenge to which anthropologically or other culturally oriented research makes a very pertinent contribution. The summary point is that basic research in culture and mental health and practical developments as illustrated for Indonesia have developed quite independently. Circumstances bring these two areas of activities into close potential articulation. Ethnomedically oriented research can make practical contributions as well as contributions to the academic disciplines that contribute concepts and theory. Among the benefits of broadened approach may be the opportunity to gain a wider critical forum and the need to design research so that results can be communicated to others in a form that transcends narrower disciplinary preoccupations.

REFERENCES

Carstairs, G. M., & Kapur, R. L. (1976). *The great universe of kota.* Berkeley: University of California Press.

Caudill, W. (1958). *The psychiatric hospital as a small society.* Cambridge, MA: Harvard University Press.

Colfer, C. (1979). *In defense of many paths.* Unpublished master's thesis, School of Public Health, University of Hawaii, Honolulu.

Connor, L. (1982). Ships of fools and vessels of the divine: Mental hospitals and madness, a case study. *Social Science and Medicine, 16,* 783-794.

Dipojono, B. (1972). Javanese mystical groups. In W. Lebra (Ed.), *Transcultural research in mental health.* Honolulu: University Press of Hawaii.

Dipojono, B. (1979a, December). Factor^2 sosio-budaya pada pengabatam tradisional orang jawa. *Simposium Kesehatan Jiwa.* Yaysan Kesehatan Jiwa Dharmawangsa dan Harian Umum Snar Harapan di Jakarta.

Dipojono, B. (1979b). *Proceedings of the Conference on Javanese Traditional Medicine and Medical Care.* Jakarta.

Directorate of Mental Health, Ministry of Health, Jakarta, Indonesia (Ed.). (1978). *Proceedings, first ASEAN teaching workshop on culture and mental health.* Unpublished manuscript.

Directorate of Mental Health, Ministry of Health, Jakarta, Indonesia (Ed.). (1979). *Proceedings, mental health technique seminar on traditional healing with specific reference to its psycho-social-cultural mechanisms.* Unpublished manuscript.

Edgerton, R. (1969) On the recognition of mental illness. In S. Plog & R. Edgerton (Eds.). *Changing perspectives in mental illness.* New York: Holt, Rinehart & Winston.

Fabrega, H. (1977a). Effects of disease as behavior: Analysis of Latino medical beliefs. *Ethos, 5,* 119-137.

Fabrega, H. (1977b). Group differences in the structure of illness. *Culture, Medicine and Psychiatry, 1,* 379-394.

Foster, G. (1977). Medical anthropology and international health planning. *Social Science and Medicine, 11,* 527-534.

Fox, R. C. (1959). *Experiment perilous.* New York: Free Press.

Gaines, A. (1979). Definitions and diagnoses: Cultural implications of psychiatric help-seeking and psychiatrists' definitions of the situation in psychiatric emergencies. *Culture, Medicine and Psychiatry, 3,* 381-418.

Geertz, C. (1960). *The religion of Java.* New York: Free Press.

Good, B. (1977). The heart of what's the matter—The semantics of illness in Iran. *Culture, Medicine and Psychatry, 1,* 25-28.

Good, B., & Good, M.J.D. (1981) The meaning of symptoms. In L. Eisenberg & A. Kleinman (Eds.), *The relevance for social science of medicine.* Dordrecht, Netherlands: Reidel.

Goris, R. (1957). The Balinese medical literature. *Djawa, 17,* 281-290.

Higgenbotham, H. (1979) Culture and the development of psychological services in developing nations. *Transcultural Psychiatric Research, 16,* 7-27.

Hirokoshi-Roe, H. (1979) Mental illness as a cultural phenomenon: Tolerance and therapeutic process among the Moslem Sudanese in West Java. *Indonesia, 28,* 121-138.

Iskandar, P., & Rienks, A. S. (1981). *Primary and indigenous health care in rural central Java: A comparison of process and contents.* Paper presented at the IVAES Congress, Amsterdam.

Kalangie, N. (1980). *Contemporary health care in a West Javanese village: The roles of traditional and modern medicine.* Unpublished doctoral dissertation, University of California, Berkeley.

Katz, M., Sanborn, K. O., Lowerey, H. A., & Ching, J. (1978). Ethnic studies in Hawaii: On psychopathology and social deviance. In L. Wynne, R. Cromwell, & S. Matthysoe (Eds.), *The nature of schizophrenia: New approaches to research and treatment.* New York: Joyhn Wiley.

Kleinman, A. (1978). International health care planning from an ethno-medical perspective: Critique and recommendations for change. *Medical Anthropology, 2*(2), 71-96.

Kleinman, A. (1980). *Patients and healers in the context of culture.* Berkeley: University of California Press.

Koentjaraningrat, R. (1979). Javanese magic, sorcery, and numerology. *Masyarakat Indonesia, 6,* 37-52.

Kraeplin, E. (1904). Vergleichende Psychiatrie. *Centralblatt fur Nerven heikundige Psychiatrie, 27* 433-437, 468-469.

Lapuz, L. (1973). *A study of psychopathology.* Quezon City: University of the Philippines Press.

Lebra, W. (1976). Culture-bound syndromes, ethnopsychiatry and alternative therapies. In *Mental health research in Asia and the Pacific* (Vol. 4). Honolulu: University Press of Hawaii.

Leimena, S. L., & Thong, D. (1979) Traditional therapeutics in Bali. In Directorate of Mental Health, Ministry of Health, Jakarta, Indonesia (Ed.), *Proceedings, mental health teaching seminar on traditional healing with specific reference to its psycho-social-cultural mechanisms.* Unpublished manuscript.

Lock, M. (1980). *East Asian medicine in urban Japan.* Berkeley: University of California Press.

Maretzki, T. (1979) Anthropology and mental health: Reflections on interdisciplinary growth. *Culture, Medicine and Psychiatry, 3*(3), 95-110.

Maretzki, T. (1981). Culture and psychopathology in Indonesia. *Transcultural Psychiatric Research Review, 18,* 237-256.

Marsella, A. (1979). Cross-cultural studies of mental disorders. In A. J. Marsella, R. Tharp, & T. Ciborowski (Eds.), *Perspectives on cross-cultural psychiatry.* New York: Academic.

Marsella, A. (1980) Depressive experience and disorder across cultures. In A. J. Marsella, H. Triandis, & J. Draguns (Eds.), *Handbook of cross-cultural psychiatry: Vol. 6. Psychopathology.* Boston: Allyn & Bacon.

Marsella, A., & Pedersen, P. (1981). *Cross-cultural counseling and therapy.* Elmsford, NY: Pergamon.

Martono, H., & Heerjan, S. (1980). *The community mental health development board of Jakarta* (Badan Pembins Kesehatan Jiwa Masyarakat DKI Jakarta). Jakarta: Jakarta Metropolitan Health Service.

Martono, H., Heerjan, S., & Harahap, A. T. (1980). *Operational plan 1981-85 of the mental health development centre.* Jakarta: Jakarta Metropolitan Health Service.

McCauley, A. P. (1979) *Preliminary report and study of the use of modern and traditional medicine in a Balinese village.* Unpublished manuscript, University of California, Berkeley.

Murphy, J., & Leighton, A. (1965). Native conceptions of psychiatric disorder. In J. M. Murphy & A. H. Leighton (Eds.), *Approaches to cross-cultural psychiatry.* Ithaca, NY: Cornell University Press.

Pfeiffer, W. (1971). *Transkulturelle Psychiatrie: Ergebnisse und Problem.* Stuttgart: Georg Thieme Verlag.

Salan, R., & Maretzki, T. W. (in press). Mental health services and traditional healing in Indonesia: Are the roles compatible? *Culture, Medicine and Psychiatry.*

Sampoerno, D. (1980). *Program kesehatan jiwa dan pendidikan kesehatan jiwa pada akhli kesehatan masyarakat di indonesia.* Paper presented at the Second National Congress to Neurology, Psychiatry and Neurosurgery, Bandung, Indonesia.

Santoso, R. (1959). The social conditions of psychotherapy in Indonesia. *American Journal of Psychiatry, 113,* 798-800.

Setyonegoro, K. (1964). Development of psychiatry in Indonesia. *Madjalah Kedokteran Indonesia, 14*(9), 8-12.

Setyonegoro, K. (1980). *Pengembangan kesehatan jiwa Indonesia segara nasional dan regional.* Paper presented at the Second National Congress of Neurology, Psychiatry and Neurosurgery, Bandung, Indonesia.

Subroto, B. (1979). The role of traditional medicine in Indonesia: A country report. In Directorate of Mental Health, Ministry of Health, Jakarta, Indonesia (Ed.), *Proceedings, mental health teaching seminar on traditional healing with specific reference to its psycho-social-cultural mechanisms.* Unpublished manuscript.

Suparlan, P. (1978). The Javanese Dukun. *Masyarakat Indonesia, 5,* 195-216.

Thong, D. (1980). *Psychiatry in the Pacific: The task of becoming.* Paper presented at the Second Pacific Congress of Psychiatry, Manila.

Townsend, J. (1978). *Cultural conceptions and mental illness.* Chicago: University of Chicago Press.

van Wulfften-Palthe, P. M. (1948). *Neurologie en Psychiatrie.* Amsterdam: Wetenschappelijke Uitgeverij.

Waxler, N. (1977). Is mental illness cured in traditional societies? A theoretical analysis. *Culture, Medicine and Psychiatry, 1,* 233-253.

World Health Organization. (1978). *Alma ata: Primary health care.* Geneva: Author.

10

BELIEF AND BEHAVIOR
IN HAITIAN FOLK HEALING

ERIKA BOURGUIGNON

INTRODUCTION

The purpose of this chapter is to discuss the role of possession belief and possession trance in Haitian folk healing. The chapter reviews various patterns of belief and ritual and their functional relationship to Haitian conceptions of personality and health.

Vodou: An Afro-American Folk Religion

In the context of the current widespread interest in traditional healing methods, *voduo,* the folk religion of Haiti, holds a special place. This syncretic religion, which combines African, Catholic, and local elements in its beliefs and rituals, has long fascinated observers. As a result, we have many descriptions and discussions of vodou, written from various points of view, some dating back to the colonial period of the eighteenth century. Although there has been substantial agreement on a core of basic facts, it is interesting to see how the diverse vantage points of the observers have tended to influence their reports. Vodou has often been decried as devil worship, paganism, or "dangerous African superstitions." In the 1920s, while their country was under U.S. occupation, some Haitian intellectuals began to develop a curiosity about folk traditions and their origins, and even a pride in their African roots. This is most clearly expressed in the writings of the Haitian physician Jean Price-Mars (1928/1973) and in the warm reception given to the work of the

American anthropologist M. J. Herskovits (1937). Yet even Price-Mars wrote of vodou as a "very primitive religion." Bastien (1966, p. 40) has remarked that "attitudes about vodou have varied with the political fortunes of Haiti." In the early 1960s, transcultural psychiatrists began to consider vodou cult leaders as traditional healers (Kiev 1961a, 1961b; Wittkower, Douyon, & Bijou, 1964).

Possession Trance

This variation in attitudes toward vodou has been paralleled by the diversity of interpretations accorded ritual possession trance, the central and most spectacular feature of vodou religion. There was, first of all, the opinion that such behavior gave evidence of a demonic presence requiring exorcism. This view is still held by fundamentalist Protestants, who have made great inroads in Haiti during the last quarter century, encouraged to some extent by the Duvalier regimes. Some of the Catholic clergy nowadays take a more ecumenical view (Conway, 1978). Second, there was the medical opinion, expressed most forcefully by J. C. Dorsainvil (1931), Haitian physician and historian. Influenced by the French psychiatric tradition, he saw possession trance as a sign of the Haitians' hereditary mental instability. His views were counterd by those of M. J. Herskovits (1937, 1949), who argued for its cultural normality, considering possession trance in the framework of cultural learning and of the African tradtion to which it clearly belongs.

Divergences in the assessment of possession trance behavior have continued to the present and are based as much or more on the differences in theoretical stance as on variations in the details of observation. Thus Alfred Metraux (1959, p. 120), in his massive study of voodoo in Haiti, writes:

> The symptoms of the opening phase of trance are clearly psychopatho-logical. They conform exactly, in their main features, to the stock clinical conception of hysteria. People possessed start by giving an impression of having lost control of their motor systems.

Metraux (1959) saw this lack of control, together with some other features of the cult, as evidence of a degeneration of the African tradition. Larose (1977, pp. 86-87) observed the same behavior, but, viewing it from the perspective of British structuralist anthropology, he offers quite a different interpretation.

These hysterical fits, deplored by Metraux as signs of anarchy, are *simply* traditional means by which the cleavage between the sacred and the profane are expressed. This cleavage has to be overdramatised in the absence of explicit rules by which religious authority is transmitted and religious power controlled: there is a need to convince, to persuade by extravagant gesture, which is not a sign of degeneration but an attribute of the system itself.

To make sense of the phenomenon of Haitian possession trance, the role it plays in the folk interpretation of mental illness and in folk methods of healing, we must consider it in a wider frame of reference. That is, we must see Haitian possession trance as only one example of a characteristic feature of African and Afro-American religions. These, in turn, are only one series of religions in the world as a whole that make use of the human capacity or propensity for possession trance. The Haitian case, then, loses the aura of the bizarre and the aberrant that it has for so many observers.

In such a comparative perspective, possession trance becomes less odd a phenomenon and, at the same time, requires more complex interpretation than any either/or position would have us believe. Explanations in the literature range from hysteria and epilepsy to cultural learning, hypnosis, and transmarginal inhibition. The behavior is clearly dissociational in nature; quite as clearly it contains a substantial component of learning. In given instances, possession trance may be pathological or therapeutic, prophylactic or theatrical. Personal motivation plays its role, but on any specific occasion, ritual and even entertainment features may predominate over personal ones. Individual needs and collective ritual demands may represent different, sometimes complementary, at times even conflicting requirements. The nature of "value" of a particular instance of possession trance must depend on the individual and the specific situation.

What I am here calling "possession trance" is generally spoken of in the French-language literature as possession "fit" or "attack" (*crise de possession*), on the analogy of a hysterical or epileptic fit.[1] It consists of an observable alteration of an individual's demeanor, and, inferentially at least, of the person's consciousness as well. It is of variable duration but generally lasts no more than several hours at a time—often much less, only rarely longer. It is this altered state that the words "trance" and "fit" (*crise*) refer to. On the other hand, in the view of the actors themselves and of others who share their outlook, the changes in behavior and experience are attributed to the presence of a spirit entity who, it is believed, has taken over the individual's ego functions—that is, has taken temporary "possession" of the human being. The altered state of consciousness serve to authenticate, for actor and observer alike, the enactment of an alternate personality.

Before dealing with the subject of possession trance in the context of Haitian vodou, it will help us to look briefly at the country and its people, at the belief system that forms the background and context of the behavior, and at the relationship between these and the folk classification of illness. My discussion is based on aspects of my own fieldwork and on observations scattered throughout the literature.

THE SETTING: HAITI

Haiti is the poorest country in the Western Hemisphere and one of the poorest in the world. More than 80% of the poeple are estimated to live on less than $100 a year. With more than 5.5 million people, the country is overpopulated (U.S. Bureau of the Census, 1980). In spite of high fertility (a birthrate of 37 per 1000 women of childbearing age) the growth rate is slowed to 2.2% by a very high rate of infant mortality, which is variously estimated at from 147 to 180 per 1000 births (Thomas 1979). The survival of their children is obviously a constant and very real concern of parents. Various health surveys have shown widespread malnutrition, particularly among children (Jelliffe & Jelliffe, 1961; Beghin, Fougère, & Kendall, 1970)[2] and lactating mothers (Wiese, 1976), and, among other endemic diseases, a high incidence of tuberculosis with inadequate utilization of treatment facilities, even when these are potentially available (Wiese, 1974). With regard to mental health, the first and only modern psychiatric treatment facility was established in 1959 with international assistance. Prior to that time, there was only a single psychiatrist in the country, working in private practice. An abandoned American military camp served as an asylum for a small number of patients.

The general language is Creole, although the official language is French. In spite of several attempts there exists no standard orthography of Creole and the vast majority of the population is illiterate. The cultural traditions, as well as the Creole language, represent a remarkable blend of African and European, particularly French, elements. The official majority religion is Catholicism, which, for the peasants and the urban poor, is intimately blended with the Afro-Catholic tradition of vodou.

VODOU

Vodou is one of a series of Afro-Catholic religions to be found in the region extending from Cuba to southern Brazil. These syncretic religions grew up during the period of slavery wherever Catholicism and African traditions met. They continue to be in a state of flux, changing as conditions demand and opportunities arise. Seen from this point of view, vodou constitutes historic psychocultural adaptation, utilizing materials from two cultural mainstreams: the European Catholic and the West African. Vodou is not only a religious system involving rituals of worship, it is also a system of dealing with practical problems, of which illness, infant mortality, and madness make up a significant part. However, at present vodou is only one of several systems people switch to in their search for help. These include traditional practices of the herbalist and home remedies, Protestantism, and scientific medicine. For the great majority of the Haitian people, the beliefs, rituals, and experiences associated with vodou provide a system of explanation, of defense in a hostile world, and a means of striving for two difficult goals: health and wealth.

The Elements of Vision

Elements of Catholic belief and ritual have been integrated into vodou. The Christian God (*Bon Dieu*) presides over the world. In more immediate contact with the faithful are three types of spirit entities: the saints (or *loa*), the dead, and the twins. All of these make ritual demands. It is the loa, however, who are believed to participate directly in the ceremonies by "possessing" their servants, or, as the Haitians say, by "mounting" their "horses." In folk belief, the human being consists of a body and two spirit entities, a "big good angel" and a "little good angel." The terminology, patterned after the idea of a guardian angel, appears both French and Catholic, but the concept of multiple souls is, in fact, of African origin.[3] The big good angel, Haitians say is displaced by the loa, who "mounts" the human being. This soul stuff may be withdrawn from the body at other occasions as well—placed into a pot for protection by the vodou priest during cult initiation, but also stolen and bottled by a sorcerer. It is this portion of the personality that is believed a sorcerer may capture immediately after death to make a *zombie,* a soulless slave.

The cult of the loa, the dead, and the twins is presided over by a vodou priest (*houngan*) or priestess (*mambo*). In rural areas the services follow family traditions and individuals acquire their duties to the spirits through inheritance from their parents. Cult practices, in this way, are tied to family lands. In urban areas (this means primarily the capital city), an individual may join a cult group, or society, headed by a priest or priestess; new quasi-kinship ties are formed under such circumstances.

As already mentioned, the world view of vodou includes many ancestral African elements, such as the concern with the dead and the twins, the inheritance of family spirits, belief in multiple souls, and the practice of ritual possession trance. Even the reference to "mounting" and "horses" in this context is African in origin. There are, however, also clearly Haitian contributions to the system: for example, the practice of inheriting spirits from both sides of the family, as land and other property are inherited under Haitian law. Also, there are many spirits of local origin and, indeed, new spirits are continuously added to the pantheons of specific individuals. (It must be remembered that not all families, or even individual family members, serve the same spirits.) Moreover, the spirit world reflects Haitian social structure, with its hierarchical arrangements of classes and color distinctions. These are evidenced in the ways in which the spirits are visualized and their roles acted out, including their physical and cultural attributes: clothes, tastes in food and drink, personal preferences and habits, language used, and so on. The spirits, it should be stressed, are highly individualized in their characteristics and in their typical behavior.

The Role of Diversity in Religion

The religious system is an open one into which new ideas and practices are constantly introduced. The great local and personal diversity in religious practice is based on the familial aspects of the religious system and on the absence of any ideological or organizational centralization. It is consistent with the general diversity in Haitian culture, which is at least in part due to the fact that Haiti is a predominantly rural country. Most of the population is dispersed throughout the countryside. Much variation is shown in language and general culture as well as in the religious sphere.

One implication of such diversity is that, beyond certain major outlines, it is not possible to describe a single system of religious beliefs and ritual practices. Each specialist can justify his or her own originality or peculiarities by reference to personal revelations from a spirit mentor. This applies to practices of diagnosis and healing as well as to other aspects of the religious and magic arts.

The Ethos of Suspicion

However, religious diversity is related to one additional factor as well. In Haiti, as elsewhere in the Caribbean region,[4] there exist what might best be termed an "ethos of suspicion,"[5] a generalized fear of others. Consequently, there is little sharing of ritual practices or of ritual knowledge that represents power. The mistrust is such that fathers will pass only a portion of their ritual knowledge on to their sons.[6]

There is a high level of insecurity in the economic realm and in the area of health. Yet peasants have very limited technical means for overcoming the dangers that face them. Under such circumstances, others are seen as major competitors for the limited good[7] that is available. The level of suspicion in interpersonal relations is high and is intimately related to a fear of magic. Much of this is believed to be wielded by specialists, whose help can be purchased. Also, numerous magically powerful groups are thought to be active under the cover of night. The world is seen as full of hostile and envious people, who do not show their true faces. Aggression by means of magic is covert. Overt expressions of aggression are carefully channeled to those lower on the status hierarchy: Children and animals are beaten in rage. In the context of vodou, women are often possessed by powerful, aggressive male spirits.

The ethos of suspicion and the resulting ambiguity in human relations are nicely illustrated in the following three citations from informants (Bourguignon, unpublished fieldnotes). Note that the ambiguity resides in human interactions and that the medium of these interactions is food (on occasion, it may also be money). The first is a statement by a young peasant woman:

> You never know who a person is. Like, a person you don't know asks for
> charity. A beggar asked a woman for some water and she chased him
> away. A second woman gave him water in a dirty pot. That poor man
> really was the Good Lord [Bon Dieu]. He told the woman there would
> be a great disaster and she should go away and not even turn around.
> Then there was a great disaster. You heard about it? That was in the
> Dominican Republic. But the woman turned around and turned into
> a rock.

Here the missionary influence is clear. The injunction to help the
least of the poor is combined with the account of Lot's wife and the
report of a real-life disaster in a neighboring country. Yet the
prefatory statement puts the story in its rightful place: "You never
know who a person is."

If it is dangerous to refuse to give charity, it is also dangerous to
comply with such a request, as is shown in another example by the
same informant:

> There is a woman or a man who seems poor, who asks for charity. You
> give her [him] 5 cents. When you go through the gate, you fall indis-
> posed. You understand that it was not a poor person.

"Falling indisposed" is a subject to which we shall return. The
disguise of beggar, it is to be understood, was assumed by an enemy
with magical powers to cause harm to the victim. Yet, if it is
dangerous both to give and not to give, it is also dangerous to take, as
seen in the following words by a young man:

> If a person gives you something to eat and you get sick, you tell your
> parents who did it before you die so they will know who killed you and
> get the government to arrest that person.

Food may be set out as the crossroads for magical purposes, for
example, to send sickness from one person to another. The person
who picks it up, it is believed, takes the sickness and thereby removes
it from the patient.[8] This was done, for example, in the case of a young
woman suffering from tuberculosis. Yet, as her brother explained, she
died anyway. Note that what is carried out as curative magic, from the
point of view of the patient, is hostile magic from the perspective of
the victim. Clearly, the implication is that health is a limited good, so
that if one person is to be free of illness, another must take it on.

Food may be placed under trees or at shrines as offerings for spirits. People who take some of it may expect to be punished. Metraux (1953) reports on several cases in which taking food from such offerings was identified by a vodou priest as the cause of death: a man who died after being kicked by his mule, another who died after a short unidentified illness in spite of the sacrifices prescribed by the vodou priest.

DIAGNOSIS IN VODOU

This last example suggest that the ritual specialist defines and, where possible, shapes the situation that is presented to him or her. As a diagnostician, he or she labels and thus identifies the behavior, putting it within the framework of familiar categories from which rituals of therapy flow. The rituals of diagnosis involve consulting the spirits, with whom the priest or priestess has special relations. They are made to speak through the specialist (in possession trance), or are called into a jar, there to speak, or through a variety of other divinatory paraphernalia. In any given case, however, the diagnostician will be influenced by the facts of the case as he or she knows them: the presenting behavior of the patient or client, the accounts given by relatives or others involved in the incident, the knowledge he or she has of the people concerned, in particular whether they are members of his or her family or cult group or are strangers, that is, nonkin or nonmembers. The therapeutic specialties of the priest or priestess and, in the city, perhaps the relations he or she entertains with a physician may also play a role.

A Case Example

A woman in her twenties told me that as a small child she was once frightened by the appearance of a large number of small snakes. The vodou priest who was consulted explained that the snakes were the spirits of the twins come to punish her for having taken some of the food offerings presented to them. She thought the priest, her uncle, had seen the snakes, although her parents had not. She told the story as illustrating her early contacts with spirits, in this case in the form of a visionary experience. She also wanted to explain that the twins can appear in the form of snakes, to show that it is dangerous to take what belongs to the spirits, and, most importantly, to demonstrate the priest's skill at discovering the source of trouble and setting things right. We cannot tell from this account how old the child was, whether she really remembered taking the food, or what the presenting symptoms were besides fright. It is tempting to think that this may well have been a convulsive episode. In any event. the priest was able to calm both the child and the parents by his definition of the situation, his admonitions, and, we may suppose, the ritual atonement he imposed. The memory, in any event, was a lasting one.

Diagnosis as a Socialization Force

Diagnosis not only serves to identify the illness but utilizes it as a form of supernatural sanction, revealing the patient's infractions and their consequences to all those who learn about the case. Consequently, illness and diagnosis are used as socializing agents, as they are in many other traditional societies.[9] The healer's failure then becomes socially as valuable as his or her success: It announces the power of the spirits and of human magicians, whose effects are possible only with the support of their spirits and through the refusal of the patient's spirits to help him or her. Over and over again one hears of magic so strong that no treatment could be found to combat it.

According to Haitian traditional theory, illness, including madness, may be due to acts of God (*maladie Bon Dieu*), to punishment by the spirits, or to magic attacks by humans. In the first case nothing can be done, except perhaps to consult a physician or convert to Protestantism. In the case of spirit anger or human malevolence, however, the vodou priest can help. There is a great reluctance to define disorders as due to acts of God in regard to which the vodou practitioner is powerless. Even in cases of tuberculosis, as we have seen, an attempt may be made to approach the disease through magical means. Over and over again, people speak of someone who "died without being sick," that is, suddenly by magic, although, in point of fact, many types of treatment had been tried, including conversion to Protestantism both by the patient and other family members, and even surgical operations in the government hospital.

CASE EXAMPLES OF MENTAL ILLNESS
IN HAITIAN CULTURAL CONTEXT

In speaking about mental illness in theory, peasants say that madness is sent as punishment by the spirits. However, when specific cases are discussed, magic is mentioned more frequently. The discovery of the cause, or causes, of the illness is linked directly to the curative process. In the case of magic, however, revenge often appears to be as important as the cure. Here are some examples:

Example 1: A young peasant woman was pointed out as an example of one who was mad. She had been beautiful and had had many suitors. When she chose one, others made magic against her, and that is how she came to be mad. She is less mad now, her head has cooled. She had a child but does not know who its father is. When a woman died of tuberculosis, she went to the wake and said she was glad because now she would get some old clothes. People know she is mad so they did not take offense. She talks to herself but what she says makes no sense. (Bourguignon, unpublished fieldnotes)

Comment: There is no mention here of any attempt at a cure. the condition is chronic, has apparently lasted for several years, but had a sudden onset. Magic is said to "heat" the victim's blood, which rushes to the head. When the head cools, the patient becomes calm. The magic is attributed to jealousy. The community forms a consensus concerning the cause and condition of the victim. There is a high degree of tolerance of chronic mental illness in rural Haiti, as long as the patients can meet their own minimal needs and do not interfere with others.

Example 2: A man is in treatment by a vodou priest, but has not been cured. He explained that he had attempted to join a society of witches in community in an attempt to make money. He was accepted and sworn to secrecy, and to seal the bargain he was served a dish of food. In it, he found human remains.[10] Frightened, he returned home and told what he had found. The witches then knew that he had revealed their secret, came to beat him and drove him mad. Informant added: "If he had kept the secret, they would not have driven him crazy. When you see a person at night [and] he asks you if you recognize him, you say 'no.' If you say 'yes,' you might lose your life." (Bourguignon, 1959, p. 38)

Comment: This is a cautionary tale, whose moral is: Don't trust strangers. Be discreet. There is no criticism of the man who wanted to join witches, who are motivated by the desire for gain. Food is the medium of human relations, even with witches. Vodou priests provide treatment, but the witches are so powerful that their victims may not be able to find a cure. This does not discount the ability of the priest and of the spirits he or she works with. Rather, it emphasizes the great and dangerous power of the witches. Also, it is probably a realistic assessment of the limited success rate of vodou priests. It is therefore in their interest to stress the power of the forces they are asked to overcome. If the cure is successful, the reputation of the healer can only be enhanced.

Note that in this example, none of the following are treated as delusional: (1) the attempt to seek out the witches, (2) the cannibal feast, (3) the witches' knowledge of events at a distance, or (4) their revenge.

Example 3: Mars (1947, pp. 105-107) reports his observation of a patient at the Beudet asylum. The patient, a 66-year-old peasant, is an alcoholic suffering from persecutory delirium. He claims to have fought for several years against a society of werewolves, headed by one of his uncles. He knows the identity of other members of the society. They seek to harm him in many ways, but he claims to be invulnerable because he wears protective amulets. He has suffered at various times from terrible dreams of persecution from his enemies. Also, they cause the ground to tremble under his feet to make him fall so they can eat him. The werewolves know his thoughts when he thinks about his affairs and repeat them out loud.

Comment: It is not known how the patient came to be committed to the asylum. It is interesting to see how much cultural material is integrated into his delusions. The existence of werewolves and amulets are part of the cultural repertory. In his home community he might well have been thought to have been driven mad by the werewolves.

A powerful and widely feared form of magical attack, causing deadly illness or madness, is described by an informant in the following discussion of a hypothetical case.

Example 4: Two people might have a quarrel, like Louis and Paul. Well, Paul would go to a sorcerer and would explain [the situation] to him, and the sorcerer would send a dead person against Louis. Then Louis would fall ill, and thrash about and tear his clothes. If Louis's mother were then to go to a sorcerer, he would find out for her that it was a dead person [who caused this illness]. And then they would take Louis to the sorcerer and the dead person would come into him and tell who had sent him and what he had been given to eat and all that. Then they would feed him. Louis would eat but actually it would be the dead person eating, and then they would send him away. Then Louis would be all right. In Jeremie [informant's home town] they don't know how to do that, so that if someone on whom a dead person had been sent were to go to Jeremie, he would have to die because they don't know how to send him away. (Bourguignon, unpublished fieldnotes).

Comment: Quarreling here is seen as leading to covert, magical attack, rather than to physical violence. Untreated madness must necessarily, in this view, lead to death. The symptoms appear to be those of great psychomotor agitation. Sorcerers act as agents to send harm, also as diviners and healers by exorcising the spirit of the dead person. The identity of the sender is sought, rather than that of the dead person, who is merely a tool, and is not seen as having a will of his own. Food is the means of attack and of removal of the harming spirit. For a young man (both Louis and Paul were teenagers), it is expected that his mother will take care of him, and this includes seeking help in a case of serious illness. To question the spirit of the dead person who is believed to have taken over the body of the patient, the sorcerer (probably a vodou priest) induces possession trance in the patient. This is necessary in order to discover the sender and the medium, that is, the specific food required. Such a possession trance is part of the cure, not part of the illness. That is, the patient's state is one of acute, disordered agitation. The possession trance that is induced imposes some order on the patient's behavior and brings it under control, prior to sending the possessing spirit away. Such a sequence of illness-causing possession and curative possession trance is to be distinguished from possession trance enacting the behavior of the spirits of the vodou cult. Metraux (1959, pp. 276-280) describes in considerable detail the spectacular treatment and cure of such a case by the mambo Lorgina. The patient's illness, however, is not identified. Lorgina often explained difficulties in curing as "complications." In the case of another patient whom I saw in her cult house, she diagnosed possession by a dead person complicated by the loa Marinette-bwa-seche (Marinette-dry-arms), a spirit of paralysis, causing a twisting of the limbs. Successful priests and priestesses may provide residential care for several patients at a time.

> *Example 5:* Mars (1947, pp. 107-112) reports the case of an 8-year-old girl, a child servant, brought to the hospital by her employer. The child, in a state of high psychomotor agitation, is terrified and claims that a magic attack has been made against her and her soul placed in a bottle in an attempt to kill her. The enemy she accuses is a vodou priest who has quarreled with her employer and had recently drunk coffee at her house. The attack was precipitated by the child's finding, early in the morning, the remains of a rooster at the door, clear evidence of magic. At one point, the child speaks of herself in the third person, saying "my horse is strong, my horse won't fall, my horse won't die for a trifle." The physician prescribes a sedative. The next day the child is normal, with no memory of the events.

Comment: The child is thrown into a state of panic by the threat—real or imagined—of a magical attack. In cultural terms, this need not be a delusion. The verbal expression of the role of the protecting spirit, who announces that his or her "horse," that is, his or her human vehicle, will not be harmed, may be interpreted as a mobilization by the child of her defenses against the danger she perceives. Such possession trance by protecting spirits, outside ritual contexts, precipitated by situations of perceived danger, are not infrequent. However, it seems unusual in one so young, for possession trance in children is rare. Note the high degree of familiarity with magic and ritual in a young child. From the point of view of the psychiatrist, this is a hysterical attack.

POSSESSION TRANCE

So far, we have seen possession trance in three quite different contexts, with different precipitating factors and different cultural evaluations: (1) possession trance by the harmful spirits of a dead person, experienced by the patient and induced for purposes of identification and exorcism; (2) possession trance experienced by the vodou priest, whose spirits are called to identify causes of illness; and (3) spontaneous possession trance by a protecting spirit, induced in a patient by acute fear.

The first of these cases involves a feared situation, possession by a dead person, but the actual possession trance is part of the cure. Possession trance by protecting spirits either in ritual situations, when they are called, as by the priest, or in crisis situations, when they spontaneously come to the rescue, is much desired. Another element that is common to these situations is the displacement of one of the souls, the big good angel, either by the dead or by the protecting spirit and, finally, in the child patient, the fear of being killed through the theft of the big good angel, placed in a bottle by the enemy. In this instance, there is a combination of an acute fear reaction and a protective possession trance. Both are considered parts of a hysterical seizure by the psychiatrist.

In the ritual context, the spirits are invited by drum rhythms, songs, and dances. Each spirit personality thus has its own particular cues that induce the possession trance.[11] This is part of the worship, the service of the spirits. Their presence is necessary for sacrifices to be effective. Moreover, it is the spirits, it is held, who heal and give advice. Consequently, in a healing ceremony, it is not necessarily the priest or priestess who goes into possession trance, but other participants in the ritual; members of the cult group or the family may have spirits speak through them. These may make demands and require ritual and secular actions as part of the healing process.

As we saw earlier, in a quotation taken from Metraux (1959), the initial phases of possession trance generally resemble hysterical attacks. The violence of a specific episode depends on a number of factors: the character of the particular spirit, the ritual mastery and esoteric knowledge of the individual, and the circumstances surrounding the particular occasion. It is generally held that each stage in the initiation process and each gain in knowledge provides increased control over the spirits, so that very powerful, elderly priests or priestesses may be seen in possession trance only rarely. On the other hand, an initial possession is expected to be disorderly, violent, and incoherent. Such initial, wild possession trances may occur among spectators at a ceremony. The presenting symptoms involve rolling about on the floor—for wild spirits cannot stand or dance—and inability to talk, so that such wild spirits cannot identify themselves. Diagnosis of the seizure as the arrival of a wild spirit will be up to the cult leader, who will be aided in the discovery of the spirit's identity by what was going on at the ceremony, the drum rhythms being played and other circumstantial evidence.

However, such seizures do often occur outside the ceremonial context as well. Haitians recognize that some people have fits or spells (la crise) that by all appearances resemble "mounting" by spirits, yet no spirit is present. Philippe and Romain (1979), who review Haitian concepts of mental illness, note that la crise refers to a number of psychiatrically distinct states for which the dominant characteristic is motor or psychic agitation. It especially denotes convulsions, hysteria, and epilepsy. Philippe and Romain (1979, p. 131) comment that, according to the patient statistics of the Mars and Kline Psychiatric Centre in Port-au-Prince (at which both authors are active),

> 50% of young girls of poor and middle class backgrounds are hysterics. The common form of hysteria in Haiti is *la grande crise,* with agitation and disordered movements of the whole body, especially the legs.

The vodou priest to whom a patient is brought must make a differential diagnosis among three possible causes: a wild spirit who wants to be established, an attack by a dead person, or, finally, a "fit" (la crise).

A wild spirit is called *bosal,* a term that was applied in colonial times to recently arrived slaves, who had not yet been baptized. A bosal spirit must be identified, and since he or she cannot speak, this identification is up to the vodou priest. A first stage of initiation involves announcing the name of the spirit and his or her special requirements, and then a "washing of the head" or "baptismal" ceremony. The spirit is established in the head, which is its permanent location, by feeding the head. In the process, the initiate comes to acquire some knowledge about the spirit, and gradually gains a degree of control, dancing and talking during possession trance at ritual occasions. Note that though it is the human subject who is untrained at the time of a first possession, it is the spirit who is considered untamed and requires control through baptism. Other spirits who may appear later are not treated in this manner and will not behave wildly. The protective spirit, the first to come, stays with the person for life, and at death must be ritually removed from the person's head.

A vodouist may have a variety of spirits, one of which is the "master of the head," the principal protective spirit. The others may come in succession and take over, depending on the ritual occasion. They will vary in behavior, reflecting what are thought to be differences in sex, personality, status, and idiosyncratic attributes. As such, they provide the individual with an array of roles outside the range of those available in daily life. Importantly, they provide an opportunity for the expression of self-assertion and aggression inappropriate to normal interpersonal relations. As I have proposed elsewhere (Bourguignon, 1965), there is evidence to suggest a continuity in motivation in spite of a discontinuity in a sense of personal identity. One might speak of a "compliant" unconscious, furthering the aims of the self. Spontaneous possession trance in crisis situations exemplifies this aspect of the phenomenon perhaps most dramatically. In this sense, possession trance is an adaptive aspect of vodou ritual practice and ideology.

In the context of a curing ritual, as already noted, several persons may experience possession trance: the patient, the ritual specialist (priest or priestess), or one or more participants, whose spirits make demands or revelations. It should be noted that the ritual specialist may not have control over such utterances and must find a way of integrating them into his or her own procedures and prescriptions.

As we have seen, from a psychiatric perspective, hysterical attacks in young girls are frequent. Also, first possessions by vodou spirits are generally said to occur in adolescents. Women by far outnumber men as possession trancers. Where a girl with the presenting symptoms of psychomotor agitation is taken, will, as a first step, affect a diagnosis. If she is taken to the vodou priest, rather than to a physician, he or she must decide whether this is indeed a first possession, an attack by a dead person, or some other magical attack on the big good angel, perhaps causing a fit (la crise). In such a case, the vodou priest has a great opportunity for structuring the incident. If the seizure is defined as due to an untamed spirit, there is no implication of pathology, in "emic" terms, as long as the appropriate rituals are performed. The person is then not considered to be a patient, but a candidate for ritual integration into a family tradition of worship.

By contrast, anyone, including adults who are cult members, may be a victim of one of the many possible forms of magical attack. A variety of symptoms, which need not be of psychiatric nature, may cause one to seek out a diviner. If a magical attack is diagnosed, the anxiety that may be assumed to be at the basis of the seizure may be relieved by the identification of the enemy responsible for the attack, the extraction of the spirit of the dead person, or the retrieval of the abducted soul. Moreover, the repressed rage that explodes in such episodes of loss of control is redirected against an enemy, often in the form of countermagic. As we saw in the case of the child servant, cited from the work of Mars (1947), a spontaneous possession trance by a protective spirit may occur in acute anxiety states. Such a mobilization of the individual's own defenses in the form of the protective spirit is likely to be encouraged by the healer.[12]

The Concept of "Soul Loss"

So far, then, we have seen that in Haitian experience seizures may occur in various cultural and psychological contexts. A spontaneous attack may be interpreted as first possession trance in a noninitiate, requiring ritual integration into the vodou cult. Alternatively, seizures may be interpreted as magical attacks, either by means of a dead person or through the abduction of the big good angel.

In addition to the "fit" (la crise), there are two other locally recognized disorders that are associated with soul loss and that, if they do not respond to home remedies, require more drastic ritual intervention. These disorders are *indisposition* and *sezi,* or sudden fright.

Philippe and Romain (1979) have studied indisposition, which they consider to be a Haitian "ethnic disorder" that is very common among women. Subjects complain of a "sensation of emptiness in the chest region, dizziness and extreme weakness" (Philippe & Romain, 1979, p. 130), of falling, inability to see, and often also to hear, what goes on about them. Weidman (1979) has described a similar syndrome among Southern Blacks, Bahamians, and Cubans, as well as Haitians, in Miami. Among Southern Blacks it is called "falling out" and among Bahamians "blacking out." Philippe and Romain (1979, p. 132) note that patients often say "I feel that my big good angel is leaving."

As we saw in one of our earlier examples, indisposition may be thought of as caused by sorcery, in that instance through the medium of giving charity. Furthermore, the state is recurrent, occurs with warning, before witnesses, in crowds; also, it is said to be related to "blood problems"—anemia, loss of blood, and, as Weidman (1979) notes, "high" or "low" blood. "High blood" is defined "as blood which rises and accumulates high in the body, affecting the head and brain" (Weidman, 1979, p. 100). "Low blood" is considered blood so weak in nutritive substances that it fails to supply the head adequately. "High" here is associated with "hot" and "low" with "cold." High and hot blood must be cooled and low and cold blood must be warmed by means of oral remedies or appropriate foods (Weidman, 1979).

Underlying such explanations is a humoral view of disease, in which the body must be kept in balance between hot and cold elements.[13] As we saw in an earlier example, madness of a violent sort is also explained by the blood rising (being high) into the brain and the head heating up, whereas quiet madness results when the head "cools."

Weidman (1979) suggests that, in its chronic form, falling out ("indisposition" in the Haitian context) may be a culture-bound reactive syndrome. She also sees it as a dissociative state that is "both psycho-genic in origin and representative of a psychophysiological state of altered consciousness" (Weidman, 1979, p. 102). She adds: "Although falling-out occurs in both sacred and secular realms . . . it becomes an illness only in secular contexts" (p. 102). If this observation is applicable to the Haitian case, it may well be that some states of indisposition are reinterpreted as possession by bosal spirits and so structured into an experience of learning ritually appropriate behavior.

Sezi, or Sudden Fright

Another emically recognized disorder is called in Creole "sezi" (from French *saississement*), and refers to a state caused by surprise and sudden fear. This, too, involves a temporary soul loss, the departure of the big good angel. According to one description (Comhaire-Sylvain & Naissance, 1959) it occurs, for example, in someone who is surprised to learn of an unexpected death. Its symptoms are given as constricted throat, cold extremities, heaviness of the stomach. It requires immediate treatment, such as a special herb tea, or, in one region, a spoonful of the milk of a mother nursing a male baby and a spoonful of sugar cane syrup. In another region, Metraux (1953) reports, sezi is said to be caused not only by sudden fear and bad news but also by an excess of indignation at being victimized. Here there is a similarity to indisposition; sezi is said to be caused by the fact that the blood goes to the head, disturbing the brain, obscuring vision, and sometimes causing blindness. (This description, taken together with its stated cause, sounds rather like a violent, though unrecognized, attack of rage.)

Sezi is particularly dangerous to nursing mothers, among whom it often results from quarrels with their husbands. Under such circumstances, it is said, the milk "falls into the blood," goes to the head, and causes temporary insanity. Sezi may also lead, it is thought, to another condition, that of "spoiled" blood. This in turn may produce a variety of ailments, including pleurisy and tuberculosis, as well as skin eruptions. Sezi, moreover, may lead to a peculiar disturbance of pregnancy, called *perdition,* in which, it is believed, the fetus does not grow, so that pregnancies of up to ten years' duration are reported! This, however, is a separate and complex subject (see Murray, 1976, for a detailed discussion).

HAITIAN CONCEPTS OF PERSONALITY AND HEALTH

The Haitian conceptions of the personality and health are at the basis of these various categories of experience. They involve the head, which is the seat of the souls, the little and the big good angels. This latter entity can be displaced in several contexts: through possession by the spirits of the vodou cult, for protection in the course of initiation, and also through magical attack and in states of agitation. All involve, both conceptually, in cultural terms, as well as subjectively, a loss of control. All, therefore, leave the individual vulnerable and in need of defense. In the case of possession trance, such defense is established by building strong, positive relations with the spirits. Thus the danger of temporary soul loss is turned into a means of acquiring protection and support stronger than that which can be given by one's own big good angel. The dissociability of the personality, which is a major element in Haitian (and much African) thinking, is ambiguous in character; it is a potential asset as well as a danger.

The head, the seat of the big good angel, is also the seat of the spirits. It must be washed and fed and, at death, the spirit, who is the master of the head, must be removed. When an individual is worried, his or her head is said to be "loaded." In excitement, the head heats up; when the head cools, the individual becomes calm, also sad. The medium of heating and cooling is the life substance, blood. Conditions of the blood are involved in a variety of ailments and are affected by emotional states, such as sezi, and also by foods and tonics. Causing and curing illness involve the manipulations of these elements: the hot and cold balance, the state of the blood and its relation to the head, and, most important, the personal identity and its variable forms.

The various elements of this system are linked by one principal medium—food: food as sacrifice to the individual's own head, and to the protecting spirits and ancestors; food, together with oral medicines and tonics, to heat or cool the blood; food as magic to harm others or to free victims of illness; food to dispatch or exorcise the dead; food to establish a pact among witches; food in the form of cannibalistic attacks of werewolves; food as charity and hospitality, food as poison; food for good and for evil, and often in ways that are ambiguous. Food is offered to others, including aspects of one's own personality, and is accepted as part of an exchange: to cause others, including various spirit entities, to do one's bidding; to conciliate the angry or to cause them to refrain from doing harm. Taking food wrongfully, greedily, or foolishly causes harm. The rules of what to offer and when and how, and what to accept and what not to accept are central to ideas of intrapersonal and interpersonal balance, harmony, and well-being. Food and eating symbolize security and interpersonal control. Food serves as a weapon and means of aggression, as well as a means of establishing harmony and healing. That these themes take on such major proportions is surely no accident in a society in which the nutritional status of the majority of the population is marginal and concern over food an ever-present reality.

CONCLUSION

Haitian peasants use a variety of healing systems: folk remedies, herb doctors, vodou practitioners, Protestantism, and scientific medicine. Several of these may be used simultaneously. Their practices are often reinterpreted to fit into a world view based on a limited number of fundamental concepts. Possession belief and possession trance are to be seen as elements within a larger and more complex scheme, where ambiguity, opportunity, interpersonal suspicion, and desperate need all play their parts.

The purpose of this chapter has been to discuss the place of possession trance in Haitian folk healing. Possession trance is seen as being a part of vodou, the folk religion of Haiti. Several related concepts have been described, including spirit possession, soul loss, and sudden fright. The cultural context of possession trance was also discussed, including the role of diagnosis as a force of socialization, and the contribution of the ethos of suspicion in perpetuating possession beliefs in Haitian society. Haitian folk conceptions of personality and health and their relationship to possession trance were discussed.

NOTES

1. Rouget (1980) provides a detailed review of the uses of these and related terms in the relevant anthropological literature both in French and in English.

2. The U.S. Bureau of the Census (1980) estimates the population of Haiti in 1979 at 5.67 million, and the average annual growth rate for the period 1970-1975 at 2.3 percent.

The most comprehensive study of Haiti's present economy is by Lundahl (1979). Of particular interest is his chapter on malnutrition and disease. He reports, for 1971, for example, 52 physicians per 100,000 population for the capital and 5 per 100,000 for the rest of the country, a total of 522. In 1965-1968, 68 percent of physicians who graduated in Haiti were practicing abroad. Lundahl's (1979) carefully stated warning should be noted: "Application of public health measures or medical care without a simultaneous attack on the nutrition problem may quite conceivably have a negative impact on rural per capital incomes" (see also Trouillot, 1980).

3. Zahan (1979, p. 8) writes: "According to African thought, the human being does not possess the unity which we attribute to him; the individual psyche is not felt to be an undivided whole. Among its component principles there exists an element which allows man to 'double' himself at certain moments in his life. . . . The self normally and naturally possesses a point of fission."

4. See, for example, Beck's (1979) account of the life of an obeah man from St. Lucia. Here a witch (a "duppy woman") causes the man's wife to "come crazy," and he himself claims to have killed the witch by magical means. The account includes the very Haitian-sounding statement: "When you see a person pass in the night never call to him. You don't know what it is" (Beck, 1979, p. 196).

5. Schwartz (1973) provides an interesting discussion of a parallel example of a "paranoid ethos" in Melanesia.

6. Larose (1977) discusses this point and gives, in some detail, information on a specific case.

7. Foster (1967) has suggested the "image of limited good" as a model describing the cognitive orientation of many peasant societies. In the view of these people, the good things in life are in limited supply, and there is no way of increasing their quantity. Hence there must necessarily be conflict over their possession.

8. Prince (1964) describes the discharge ceremony of a mental patient among the Yoruba. Materials used in the ceremony are thrown into the river and carried off by the waters. Anyone picking them up, he notes, "will contract the illness" (p. 102).

9. See Hallowell (1976) for a discussion of disease and healing among the Ojibwa, where he stresses the social role of the discovery of the causes of disease.

10. Prince (1964, pp. 90-91) quotes a passage from Morton-Williams (1956), citing the confession of a member of a witchcraft society among the southwestern Yoruba: "Once they asked me to come and take soup with them. I ate it before I knew it was human flesh. . . . Until I took the soup, they said I was the sort of person likely to give away their secrets."

11. These cues are psychological in nature. No claim is made here for physiological modes of induction. See Rouget (1980) for a severe critique of claims that music has a physiological action in the induction trance states.

12. Douyon (1966) describes hysterical attacks in female adolescents in urban Haiti. He notes the occurrence of a somnambulistic state during which the patient engages in a dialogue with an imaginary presence, usually a girl friend, thus giving spontaneous expression to her thoughts and feelings. Douyon also describes, in general terms, the treatment of hysterical seizures by a vodou priest, who speaks first to a hostile spirit and then to a protective spirit, both impersonated by the patient during possession trance.

13. Wiese (1976) discusses the effect of food taboos derived from humoral medicine on the diet of lactating mothers.

REFERENCES

Adler, A., & Zempleni, A. (1972). *Le baton de l'aveugle: Divination, maladie et pouvoir chez les Mundong du Tchad.* Paris: Herman.

Bastien, R. (1966). Voudoun and politics in Haiti. In *Religion and Politics in Haiti* (ICR Studies 1). Washington, DC: Institute for Cross-Cultural Research.

Beck, J. C. (1979). *To windward of the land: The occult world of Alexander Charles.* Bloomington: Indiana University Press.

Beghin, I., Fougère, W., & Kendall, K. W. (1970). *L'alementation et la nutrition en Haiti.* Paris.

Bourguignon, E. (1959). The persistence of folk belief: Some notes on cannibalism and Zombis in Haiti. *Journal of American Folklore, 72,* 36-46.

Bourguignon, E. (1965). The self, the behavioral environment and the theory of spirit possession. In M. E. Spiro (Ed.), *Context and meaning in cultural anthropology.* New York: Free Press.

Comhaire-Sylvain, S., & J. Naissance. (1959). Mort, etat-civil a Kenskoff (Haiti). In *Revue de l'Institut de Sociologies.* Brussels.

Conway, F. J. (1978). *Pentecostalism in the context of Haitian religion and health practice.* Ann Arbor: University Microfilms.

Dorsainvil, J. C. (1931). *Vodou et nevroses.* Port-au-Prince: Imprimerie "la Presse."

Douyon, C. (1966). Les formes culturelles de l'expression de l'hysterie de conversion en Haiti. *Bulletin du Centre de Psychiatrie et de Neurologie, 5,* 26-33.

Foster, G. M. (1967). *Tzintzuntzan: Mexican peasants in a changing world.* Boston: Little, Brown.

Hallowell, A. I. (1976). Ojibwa world view and disease. In *Contributions to anthropology: Selected papers of A. Irving Hallowell.* Chicago: University of Chicago Press.

Herskovits, M. J. (1937). *Life in a Haitian valley.* New York: Knopf.

Herskovits, M. J. (1949) *Man and his works.* New York: Knopf.

Jelliffe, D., & Jelliffe, E. F. (1961). The nutrition standard of Haitian children. *Acta Tropica, 18,* 42-45.

Kiev, A. (1961a). Folk psychiatry in Haiti. *Journal of Nervous and Mental Disorders, 132,* 260-265.

Kiev, A. (1961b). Spirit possession in Haiti. *American Journal of Psychiatry, 118,* 133-151.

Larose, S. (1977). The meaning of Africa in Haitian Vodu. In I. M. Lewis (Ed.), *Symbols and sentiments: Cross-cultural studies in symbolism.* London: Academic.

Lundahl, M. (1979). *Peasants and poverty: A study of Haiti.* New York: St. Martin's.

Mars, L. (1947). *La lutte contre la folie.* Port-au-Prince: Imprimerie de l'Etat.

Metraux, A. (1953). Medicine et vodou en Haiti. *Acta Tropica, 10*, 18-68.

Metraux, A. (1959). *Vodou in Haiti.* New York: Oxford University Press.

Morton-Williams, P. (1956). The Atinga cult among the south-western Yoruba. *Bulletin de l'IFAN, 18*, 315-334.

Murray, F. G. (1976). Women in perdition: Ritual fertility control in Haiti. In J. F. Marshall & S. Polgar (Eds.), *Culture, natality and family planning.* Chapel Hill: North Carolina Population Center.

Philippe, J., & Romain, J. B. (1979). Indisposition in Haiti. *Social Science and Medicine, 13B*, 129-133.

Price-Mars, J. (1973). *Ainsi parla l'oncle* (nouvelle ed.). Montreal: Lemeac. (Original work published 1928)

Prince, R. (1964). Indigenous Yoruba psychiatry. In A. Kiev (Ed.), *Magic, faith and healing.* New York: Free Press.

Rouget, G. (1980). *La transe et la musique: Esquisse d'une theorie generale des relations de la musique et de la possession.* Paris: Gallimard.

Schwartz, T. (1973). Cult and context: The paranoid ethos in Melanesia. *Ethos, 1*, 153-174.

Thomas, J. (1979, September 2). Two countries, two approaches to population control. *New York Times*, p. E16.

Trouillot, M. R. (1980). Review of peasants and poverty: A study of Haiti by Mats Lundahl. *Journal of Peasant Studies, 8*(1), 112-116.

U. S. Bureau of the Census. (1980). *World population 1979: Recent demographic estimates for the countries and regions of the world.* Washington, DC: Government Printing Office.

Weidman, H. (1979). Falling out: A diagnostic and treatment problem viewed from a transcultural perspective. *Social Science and Medicine, 13B*, 95-112.

Wiese, H. J. (1974). Tuberculosis in rural medicine. *Social Science and Medicine, 8*, 359-362.

Wiese, H. J. (1976). Maternal nutrition and traditional food behavior in Haiti. *Human Organization, 35*(2), 193-199.

Wittkower, E. D., Douyon, L., & Bijou, L. (1964). Spirit possession in Haitian Vodun ceremonies. *Acta Psychoterhapeutica et psychosomatica, 12*, 72-80.

Zahan, D. (1979). *The religion, spirituality, and thoughts of traditional Africa.* Chicago: University of Chicago Press.

11

PSYCHOTHERAPY
A Cross-Cultural Perspective
from Japan

TAKEO DOI

This chapter attempts a cross-cultural perspective on psychotherapy. The rationale that calls for such a perspective at the present time is as follows. First, it is now widely acknowledged that all kinds of psychotherapy are deeply rooted in the culture of their origin. This can be said not only of clearly culture-bound psychotherapy, such as Morita therapy in Japan or some folk therapies in developing countries, but also of admittedly culture-free psychotherapy such as psychoanalysis. Second, because of the insight into the cultural origin of various forms of psychotherapy, a new awareness has developed of the necessity for cultural sensitivity within psychotherapy, that is to say, cross-cultural psychotherapy, particularly when the therapist and the patient do not come from the same cultural background. Third, there is, nonetheless, a seemingly opposite trend to this new awareness, since certain originally esoteric forms of psychotherapy may find a clientele among a population that is not related to the culture of their origin. One can immediately call to mind as an example the recent vogue of transcendental meditation in certain parts of the United States. In the same vein, one may interpret the fact that Western-based psychoanalysis finds adherents in non-Western countries such as Japan or India.

This crossing of psychotherapy beyond its original cultural boundary may not be surprising, however, if one considers the facts that today, compared with previous ages, an increasing number of people are crossing from one culture to another and that cultures themselves are undergoing changes due to influences from extraneous cultures. As a matter of fact, it is not infrequent nowadays, especially in the United States, that a person coming from a completely different culture serves as psychiatrist in a host culture, or even becomes a professor of psychiatry, teaching neophytes the trade of psychotherapy. Furthermore, during the past several decades, cultural mixing has occurred at an accelerated pace at the level of culture itself as well as among various populations. This coincides significantly with the mushrooming of new brands of psychotherapy as well as the keen interest shown by various disciplines in the cultural aspects of psychotherapy (Marsella, Tharp, & Cibrowski, 1979; Lebra, 1976; Pedersen, Draguns, Lonner, & Trimble, 1981). With these factors in mind, it is all the more urgent to have a clear perspective on the relationship between psychotherapy and culture.

Before I proceed to the main points of my discussion, a few words are necessary about the type of approach I will take. I have said that this chapter offers a cross-cultural perspective on psychotherapy. I want to emphasize that it is a perspective, not an overview of all the pertinent literature on the subject. In order to have a perspective, one must ascertain where one stand vis-à-vis the particular subject one is investigating and how one came to that view, for these are the very things that decide the kind of perspective one achieves. In other words, any perspective must be personal. So, in presenting my perspective, let me briefly state my background in order to clarify the point from which I shall proceed.

THE POINT OF PERSPECTIVE

I was born in Japan and educated there through medical school, from which I graduated in 1942. I later had the good fortune to study in the United States, first for two years (from 1950 to 1952) and, after a five-year interval, for yet another year. Prior to this, I was already interested in the psychological problems the patients almost invariably presented in my medical practice during the postwar years. At the time, I did not know what to do with them, since I had been taught nothing about them in my medical education. So I avidly read as many articles in American journals as I could obtain that dealt with such problems as I was faced with in my practice. Naturally, I was very happy when the opportunity arose to study in the United States. It was a great learning experience for me in many ways, because it was the first time that I experienced a culture completely different from my own. What was most important for my subsequent career was the full exposure to a psychoanalytic psychiatry that was diametrically different from the prewar German school of psychiatry that I had learned in medical school.

At that time, psychoanalysis was at the peak of its popularity in the United States. Actual exposure to this fact aroused my curiosity as to why psychoanalysis was so popular in the United States, apparently more so than in Europe where it originated, and also made me wonder why it did not fire fervor in Japan, for Freud's ideas had been introduced through the Japanese translation of his main works in the early part of this century. My attention was also called to Morita therapy as a unique Japanese psychotherapy and I was struck by a peculiar difference between this and psychoanalysis, not only in terms of therapeutic procedures or theories behind them, but what these two regarded as suitable cases for their treatment methods. Psychoanalysis began with treatment of hysterical cases, whereas Morita therapy began with hypochondriacal cases. Each specifically regarded as unsuitable for its treatment method that which the other regarded as suitable. At least, those were Freud's and Morita's positions, respectively, when they began their work.

These questions have haunted me and still do to a certain extent. It was in grappling with these questions that my own theory of *amae* was developed; I have written a great deal about amae both in Japanese and English (Doi, 1962, 1963, 1973a). I shall mention a few points here that directly concern the questions I raised above. First, for Japanese people as a whole, dependency need is readily admitted to one's consciousness as well as subjected to control by the kind of interpersonal relationships one enters, while for Americans it seems to be altogether repressed or denied. On the one hand we find among Japanese the existence of a unique concept of amae denoting the satisfaction of such a need and a related vocabulary to describe its manifestations in various situations, including its frustration; among Americans, on the other hand, we find the idealization of individual freedom and independence.

Second, it was perhaps because it catered to the wish to determine one's own destiny that psychoanalysis became popular in the United States, for, according to its doctrines, one controls one's destiny by mastering one's unconscious. Thus psychoanalysis helps promote in the minds of those who engage in it the precious illusion of control over fate, that is, the sense of autonomy. In Japan, on the other hand, it could never have hoped to become popular precisely because in the Japanese ethos one is taught always to take into account fate, which shapes one's destiny. Undoubtedly, this difference in attitudes toward fate is related to the difference in the attitudes toward dependency need. One may say that dependency need by definition all but precludes autonomy, for it is contingent for its satisfaction on so many factors one cannot control—in short, on fate.

Third, Morita therapy succeeded where psychoanalysis failed, presumably because in Morita therapy the problems of dependency are dealt with intuitively. However, it is only in recent years that psychoanalysis came to grips conceptually with these problems. It would appear that the Japanese experience concerning dependency need, in addition to being an expression of Japanese culture, can claim universal validity. In fact, it is my understanding that such a view may release psychoanalysis from its culture-specific underpinnings and strengthen it as a universal theory.

A THEORETICAL MODEL FOR PSYCHOTHERAPY

I think from the beginning my impulse has been to seek a unified theory for psychotherapy, though I have been fully aware of the existing cultural differences. This impulse has been further stimulated by the development during the past few decades of many new psychotherapeutic methods, which I suspect were the result of social and cultural changes in recent years. In short, I have wanted to bring a certain order to the chaos that has overtaken the field of psychotherapy and have sincerely thought that it would also serve the purpose of consolidating the psychiatrist's position in this expanding field. Many have attempted a similar venture, apparently with the same motive (Karasu, 1977; Neil & Ludwig, 1980; Ellenberger, 1982; Havens, 1981); mine appeared in a short paper titled "Psychotherapy as Hide-and-Seek" (Doi, 1973b), in which I proposed that the children's game of hide-and-seek, and its earlier form, peekaboo, consisting of alternate disappearing and reappearing, serves as a theoretical model for all kinds of psychotherapy, ancient and modern, Eastern and Western. It is difficult to say why I hit upon this idea. All I can say is that I must have been led to this proposition from three premises: first, that all forms of psychotherapy are based upon the interpersonal relationship; second, dependency need is instrumental in inducing the interpersonal relationship or object relations at infancy or even in later years, hence it should also underlie the psychotherapeutic relationship; third, the measure of dependency need that operates in the psychotherapeutic relationships can be adequately characterized by hide-and-seek and peekaboo.

Hide-and-seek can be played only by those children who have established object relations, whereas peekaboo is more appropriate for those who are in the process of developing object relations. In psychotherapy, the patient is urged to engage in either or both of the two following activities: namely, to explore the hidden psyche that is the cause of his or her trouble and to be reassured and comforted by the presence of the therapist on whom the patient comes to depend. It appears that the former process is hide-and-seek and the latter is peekaboo. I think this model of hide-and-seek and peekaboo for psychotherapy can be further simplified, for there is definitely a developmental continuum from peekaboo to hide-and-seek and both are based on the dichotomous pattern of familiar-unfamiliar that emerges in early infancy. This aspect of infant development has been investigated by Bowlby (1971) and others, but I shall not go into details here. It will suffice to point out that all kinds of psychotherapy take after the patterns of familiar-unfamiliar, because, just as the infant is drawn toward the familiar and avoids or is alarmed by what is strange, psychotherapy in any form attempts to make whatever threatens the patient innocuous and acceptable. Let us see in detail how this model fits in with all forms of psychotherapy.

PSYCHOTHERAPIES IN VIEW OF
THE ABOVE MODEL

I shall enumerate various kinds of psychotherapy to see if each can be explained by the above model. In psychoanalysis one has to be sufficiently secure to embark on a lonely journey, albeit with the help of the analyst, seeking a pathogenic secret in one's hidden psyche. Thus psychoanalysis is hide-and-seek within one's own person. Exploratory psychotherapy other than orthodox psychoanalysis may be included in this category. Compared to this kind of psychotherapy, supportive psychotherapy is essentially peekaboo, inasmuch as one is reassured and comforted by the presence of others, thus being strengthened and confirmed in one's vital ties with others. I think both exploratory and supportive psychotherapy can be nicely summed up by the familiar-unfamiliar pattern as was hinted above. That is, in the former the pathogenic material is pathogenic precisely because it is perceived as foreign to oneself and has to be drawn out in order to make it more to one's liking; in the latter the familiar side of personality is to be reinforced vis-à-vis the unfamiliar world.

It is interesting to note here that the conceptual distinction between explorative and supportive psychotherapy, though it may be blurred in actual practice, is peculiar to those Western societies in which the tenets of psychoanalysis are accepted. It goes without saying also that psychoanalysis in its individualistic form could develop only in the Western world. As for supportive psychotherapy, the story is a bit complicated and I shall come back to this later. Now, what I would like to emphasize here is the fact that in all non-Western psychotherapies the explorative aspect of the supportive aspect are always intermingled, that is, not separated as in Western societies. Take shamanism or religious healing, for instance. What troubles the person is divined by the shaman, a process that somewhat resembles explorative psychotherapy in the Western world. But what is noteworthy is that this act takes place usually in the public or within a setting of communal living. Particularly in primitive societies it is a rule that the whole congregation participates in the healing process, thus helping the afflicted one to be restored to his or her proper place in society. This aspect of shamanism undoubtedly corresponds to supportive psychotherapy in the Western world.

Interestingly, this blending of the explorative and the supportive also applies to Morita therapy and Naikan therapy, the methods of treatment developed in modern Japan. I shall not try to belabor this point here, since both therapies are well described in English (Kondo, 1976; Murase, 1976) and the above point is apparent to anyone who has read about those therapies. I would also like to add that the distinction between the explorative and the supportive does not apply either to behavioral or to existential therapy, though the model of psychotherapy I have proposed above applies equally to both: Namely, the learning that is so much emphasized in behavioral therapy is to make what is unfamiliar familiar and the experience that supposedly promotes personal growth in existential therapy is predicated upon the genuine familiarity shared by therapist and patient.

Therefore, the theoretical model I have proposed fits in very well with any form of psychotherapy and gives some order to so confused and fluid a field as psychotherapy. Furthermore, it solves the question of cultural varieties in psychotherapy at one stroke, for culture is what is shared by the members of a community as familiar. Naturally, it differs from culture to culture. But then the question arises as to whether or not psychotherapy is the same as culture learning, that is to say, ordinary education. Certainly, it may not be unreasonable to place psychotherapy within the broader category of education. One may note in this regard that Freud (1963) called psychoanalytic treatment a kind of after-education. But the further question arises as to why psychoanalysis and other schools of psychotherapy developed particularly in nineteenth-century Europe. Why do they still flourish and proliferate in the contemporary world? It is to these questions that I will now turn.

PSYCHOTHERAPY AND CULTURAL CONFLICTS

I shall begin by asking whether there is any special characteristic that distinguishes psychotherapy from ordinary culture learning or acculturation. The answer to this question involves the very problems of culture, because, in ordinary culture learning, culture itself is never questioned—it is taken for granted. Psychotherapy is indicated where culture itself has to be questioned, specifically, when the internalization of the conflicting cultural values disturbs one's familiar world, making one part of the self strange to another, thus leading to alienation from the self.

The internalization of the conflicting cultural values is not the same as the concept of instinctual conflict that Freud made so much use of in his theory of neuroses. However, it is possible to interpret the instructual conflict as a a result of cultural conflicts, since the instinctual conflict necessarily involves cultural values. Or, taking the instinctual conflict to be basic to psychopathology, as Freud did, one can see that the existence of conflicts resulting from the clash of different cultural values weakens the hold of the cultural regulations over instinctual drives, thus leading to the instinctual conflict. At any rate, it is logical to assume that the existence of conflicts precedes the development of psychopathology, which is the object of psychotherapy. It follows that the main task of psychotherapy is to identify whatever conflict afflicts the person, then to isolate it in order to prevent it from affecting the whole person and if possible to heal the division within the person. It think that focusing upon the conflict within the afflicted person is most deliberately dealt with in psychoanalysis and its related schools. I should think that the same process takes place inadvertently in other schools of psychotherapy as well, aht is, apart from the therapist's intention, even in behavioral and existential therapies.

Now if what distinguishes psychotherapy from ordinary culture learning lies in the preexistence of cultural conflicts, it becomes easier to answer the question of why the important schools of psychotherapy developed in nineteenth-century Europe. As van den Berg (1974) illustrates by many examples in his historical and sociocultural studies, there is no doubt that the development of modern psychotherapies is related to the profound changes in Europe during the past centuries, which culminated in disruption of its traditional unity, thus generating conflicts in various spheres of society. In this regard, one may well understand the notion of anomie formulated by Emile Durkheim. I once addressed the same question with regard to psychoanalysis in one of my papers:

> It is well to remember here, however, that at the time when psychoanalysis was first invented by Freud the cataclysm of the Western world was already under way. One can recall in this regard names like Nietzsche and Kierkegaard. Is not the development of psychoanalysis also related to this cultural and social crisis? Heinz Hartman [1958], reflecting on the question of why psychoanalysis emerged at the time it did, stated as follows: "Apparently at certain points in history the ego can no longer cope with its environment, particularly not with that which it itself has created: the means and goal of life lose their orderly relation, and the ego then attempts to fulfill its organizing function by increasing its insight into the inner world." In other words, psychoanalysis was an attmept of the ego to re-collect itself vis-à-vis the demoralizing world. (Doi, 1964, p. 13)

The above thesis, which relates the development of modern psychotherapies to historical changes, can be equally stated about the cases of Morita therapy and Naikan therapy in Japan. Both came into existence in the present century, presumably because a large number of Japanese people who were undergoing modernization and its accompanying cultural conflicts suffered from neuroses and needed special help. This is evident in Morita therapy, where the patient is repeatedly reassured of the normality and naturalness of his or her socially untoward reactions, and in Naikan therapy, where the patient is urged to recollect his or her so far unacknowledged debts to close relatives. Remember that the features emphasized in these therapies are the things that tend to be overlooked in the inhumanly competitive life of the contemporary world. It is for this reason that these therapies help the patients recover the lost balance of their minds, which initiated their mental sufferings.

Furthermore, there is good reason to believe that the folk therapies in so-called primitive societies (at least some of them) may also be a reaction to the crises caused by the intrusion of Western civilization into their world. Prince (1979) cites two examples: a new type of healing shrine among the rural Ashanti and other groups in response to the disorganizing effects of Westernization (described by M. J. Field) and the healing sessions in Iquitos by culturally mixed populations undergoing rapid culture changes. I suspect that if one examines developing countries more carefully, one may find more examples of this kind. For instance, the cargo cult in Melanesia, which has been reported since the late nineteenth century, may be another such example. This is a cult that expects the resolution of social, political, and economic problems all at once by the arrival of an imaginary cargo full of wealth. Burton-Bradley (1975, p. 16), who studies the culture extensively, states:

> Cargo anxiety is the essential feature of many instances of pathological anxiety in Melanesia. It is essentially a status anxiety which arises from imbalance between the forces making for development and those of the status quo. It is the consequence of cultural encounter. It permeates almost all aspects of life, often in covert or subdued form, and it embellishes the symptomatology of many forms of psychiatric disorder. . . . Each patient is a real or potential cargo leader, fortuitously cut short in the course of his career.

Incidentally, the same logic may be applied to the syncretistic aspects of shamanistic religions noted by various scholars. It is likely that they resulted from the efforts to cope with induced cultural changes. Thus the fact of syncretism is the historical residue of cultural changes, though the shamans, in the apt phrase of Hippler (1976, p. 103), simply "change their tactics with their cultural milieu." I assume that the same mechanism might have operated behind the famous syncretism in the ancient Mediterranean civilization as well as the similar phenomena manifested in the history of religions in Japan. To pursue this line of argument, however, would be beyond the scope of this chapter.

THE SUPPORTIVE FUNCTION OF
PSYCHOTHERAPY IN THE PRESENT AGE

When one surveys the developments in psychotherapy during the past few decades, one cannot help but be struck by an emerging emphasis on its supportive function. I think it was during the 1950s, when psychoanalysis was most prestigious and idealized in the minds of many professionals, that one began hearing about supportive psychotherapy. It was then thought of only as a second best for those cases that were not amenable to the strict psychoanalytic approach. Lately, however, this attitude has considerably changed and supportive psychotherapy has grown steadily in importance, so much so that even in psychoanalysis there is now mention of its supportive function. For this one may refer to the parental component in the analyst's identity, according to Stone (1961), or the holding environment provided by the analyst, according to Winnicott (1965). If one looks beyond the narrow confines of individual psychoanalysis, the emphasis on the supportive function of psychotherapy is too obvious to attract attention. But how else would one explain a new popularity of group psychotherapy or family therapy? The spread of the therapeutic community approach may also bespeak the same trend. More significantly, whenever the therapeutic strategy for each patient is discussed at clinical conferences, one would invariably hear whether the patient's support system is adequate or needs reinforcement. The success of "crisis intervention" hinges upon whether or not the patient's support system can be mobilized speedily and effectively.

I think this emphasis on the supportive function of psychotherapy can easily be interpreted as a response to a widely felt need in the contemporary world. In the present age, because of wars, revolutions, and unprecedented changes caused by advanced technology, many people feel increasingly insecure, dislocated, and exposed to unknown dangers, as everywhere the familiar world appears to be shrinking ever more rapidly. Terms such as "pluralism" or "cultural relativism" are only academic euphemisms; they may soothe the minds of intellectuals, but ordinary people would prefer to flock to whatever promises them protection from the unknown menace they intuitively sense. Hence the development of new therapies in both advanced and developing countries as a kind of shelter from the unfamiliar world. In this connection, it may be interesting to note the new rise in occultism or superstitious beliefs in advanced countries, which is evidence that the recognition of "fate," which had hitherto been breezily disavowed, is once again assuming a position of importance in the minds of people.

I would like to mention in passing that the character of the present age has been noticed by many perceptive people and for quite some time. Among others, I shall cite below the words of Philip Rieff (1966, p. 57), who related the birth of psychoanalysis to the present age: "Psychoanalysis is yet another method of learning how to endure the loneliness produced by culture. A tolerance of ambiguities is the key to what Freud considered the most difficult of all personal accomplishments: a genuinely stable character in an unstable time." The thought expressed in these lines is somewhat similar in sentiment to what I tried to convey in the previously quoted passage from one of my papers. At any rate, what is interesting is the fact that psychoanalysis itself, apart from its being an explorative and individualistic endeavor, seems to have had a supportive function from its very beginning.

CONCLUSION

Juris G. Draguns (1981) notes in his paper, "Counseling Across Cultures: Common Themes and Distinct Approaches," that contributions from the psychodynamic schools to cross-cultural counseling are lacking. Draguns (1981, p. 16) states: "What is the relevance for the delivery and implementation of cross-cultural counseling services of this theoretical perspective, especially of its emphasis upon intrapsychic conflict and unconscious determinants of behavior?" I think this chapter can be said to be an attempt to meet his challenge. I have tried to offer a theoretical model that can encompass all forms of psychotherapy, and I have indicated that the kind of psychopathology that becomes the object of psychotherapy invariably involves cultural values insofar as they engender psychic conflicts. I have shown that the development of modern psychotherapy in the West manifests this point.

The lesson from the above analysis is obvious. We hear often nowadays that Western psychotherapies cannot be applied to non-Western patients. It is no wonder, because Western psychotherapies presuppose the existence of cultural conflicts peculiar to Western people. As a matter of fact, even in the West the forms of psychotherapy are changing precisely because the cultural conflicts underlying psychic pathology are changing. Thus it is a known fact that the number of patients to whom the classical technique of orthodox psychoanalysis is applicable is decreasing, hence the explosion of new forms of psychotherapy in recent years. But non-Western societies are no less subject to cultural changes, particularly as a result of the thrust of Westernization. This naturally leads to cultural conflicts and thereby makes people susceptible to psychopathology, which requires the application of psychotherapeutic procedures. It is important to remember, however, that the purpose of psychotherapy in non-Western societies is not to promote Westernization; rather, it concerns the conflicts created by Westernization, but it is not the same as promoting Westernization. Psychotherapy tries to aid an otherwise failing traditional identity and strives to reintegrate, when possible, traditional values and imported ones. That is the essence of what we learn from the development of modern psychotherapies in the West.

REFERENCES

Bowlby, J. (1971). *Attachment.* London: Penguin.

Burton-Bradley, B. G. (1975). *Stone age crisis: A psychiatric appraisal.* Nashville: Vanderbilt University Press.

Doi, T. (1962). Amae: A key concept for understanding Japanese personality structure. In R. J. Smith & R. K. Beardsley (Eds.), *Japanese culture: Its development and characteristics* (pp.132-139). Chicago: Aldine.

Doi, T. (1963). Some thoughts on helplessness and the desire to be loved. *Psychiatry: Journal for the Study of Interpersonal Processes, 26,* 266-272.

Doi, T. (1964). Psychoanalytic therapy and Western man: A Japanese view. *International Journal of Social Psychiatry, 1* 13-18.

Doi, T. (1973a). *The anatomy of dependence* (J. Bester, Trans.). Tokyo: Kodansha.

Doi, T. (1973b). Psychotherapy as "hide and seek." *Bulletin of the Meninger Clinic, 37,* 174-177.

Draguns, J. G. (1981). Counseling across cultures: Common themes and distinct approaches. In P. Pedersen, J. G. Draguns, W. J. Lonner, & J. E. Trimble (Eds.), *Counseling across cultures.* Honolulu: University Press of Hawaii.

Ellenberger, H. F. (1982). Evolution of the ideas about the nature of the psychotherapeutic process in the Western world. In T. Ogawa (Ed.), *The history of psychiatry: Mental illness and its treatments* (pp. 1-26). Tokyo: Saiko.

Freud, S. (1963). Introductory lectures of psychoanalysis. In *The standard edition of the complete psychological works of Sigmund Freud* (Vol. 16, p. 451). London: Hogarth.

Hartman, H. (1958). *Ego psychology and the problem of adaptation.* New York: International Universities Press.

Havens, L. L. (1981). Twentieth century psychiatry: A view from the sea. *American Journal of Psychiatry, 138*, 1279-1287.

Hippler, A. E. (1976). Shamans, curers and personality: Suggestions toward a theoretical model. In W. P. Lebra (Ed.), *Mental health research in Asia and the Pacific: Vol. 4, Culture-bound syndromes, ethnopsychiatry and alternate therapies.* Honolulu: University Press of Hawaii.

Karasu, T. B. (1977). Psychotherapies: An overview. *American Journal of Psychiatry, 134*, 851-863.

Kondo, K. (1976). The origin of Morita therapy. In W. P. Lebra (Ed.), *Mental health research in Asia and the Pacific: Vol. 4. Culture-bound syndromes, ethnopsychiatry and alternate therapies.* Honolulu: University Press of Hawaii.

Lebra, W. P. (Ed.). (1976). *Mental health research in Asia and the Pacific: Vol. 4. Culture-bound syndromes, ethnopsychiatry and alternate therapies.* Honululu: University Press of Hawaii.

Marsella, A. J., Tharp, R., & Cibrowski, T. (Eds.). (1979). *Perspectives on cross-cultural psychology.* New York: Academic.

Murase, T. (1976). Naikan therapy. In W. P. Lebra (Ed.), *Mental health research in Asia and the Pacific: Vol. 4. Culture-bound syndromes, ethnopsychiatry and alternate therapies.* Honolulu: University Press of Hawaii.

Neil, J. R., & Ludwig. A. M. (1980). Psychiatry and psychotherapy: Past and future. *American Journal of Psychotherapy, 24*, 39-50.

Pedersen, P. B., Draguns, J. G., Lonner, W. J., & Trimble, J. E. (Eds.). (1981). *Counseling across cultures.* Honolulu: University Press of Hawaii.

Prince, R. (1979). Variations in psychotherapeutic procedures. In A. J. Marsella, R. Tharp, & T. Cibrowski (Eds.), *Perspectives on cross-cultural psychology.* New York: Academic.

Rieff, P. (1966). *The triumph of the therapeutic: Uses of faith after Freud.* New York: Harper & Row.

Stone, L. (1961). *The psychoanalytic situation.* New York: International Universities Press.

van den Berg, J. H. (1974). *Divided existence and complex society.* Pittsburgh: Duquesne University Press.

Winnicott, D. W. (1965). *The maturational process and the facilitating environment.* London: Hogarth.

12

MENTAL HEALTH SERVICES ACROSS CULTURES
Some Concluding Thoughts

NORMAN SARTORIUS
PAUL B. PEDERSEN
ANTHONY J. MARSELLA

The argument about the applicability of Western mental health concepts to other parts of the world seems to have undergone a curious reversal. While Marsella and Higginbotham have pointed out the dangers of overdependence on Westernized methods, there are also data suggesting that Westernized methods are extremely popular. Maretzki suggests that Indonesia, for example, should be allowed to incorporate Westernized methods if it so chooses. While German points out how frequently Westernized methods are criticized as "imposed" or "pseudo" etic, the continued and perhaps even increased emphasis on Westernization may be viewed as a positive as well as a negative factor. The socioeconomic climates of Third World countries often share problems with industrialized countries. "Western" influences have strongly influenced the definition of modern mental health methods. Western-originated medical technology has become more popular throughout the world and Western medicine is perceived as an alternative whenever indigenous methods fail. The Western perspective has itself changed to accommodate broader cultural perspectives in recent years.

By combining the culture-specific (emic) and culture-general (etic) viewpoints it becomes possible to see the fields of mental health in a world perspective. This larger perspective is an essential starting point for mental health professionals seeking to avoid "cultural encapsulation" by their own culture-specific assumptions. This larger perspective is also an exciting opportunity for those seeking to apply the best elements from each cultural setting in culture-general (etic) patterns that connect the various viewpoints. Each of the preceding chapters illustrates aspects of this world perspective through a "new doctrine" of mental health care that goes beyond current controversies, demonstrates the positive potential of Westernization, defines the balance of alternatives for decision making, and outlines future potentials for the fields of mental health. The world perspective goes beyond a study of exotic populations from different cultures and examines guidelines for excellence for mental health as a whole.

The chapters in this volume are concerned with the delivery of mental health services across cultural boundaries. Sections of the volume are devoted to the problems associated with the assessment and treatment of mental disorders and the training and education of professionals providing these services. These complex issues can be raised but not solved by this introductory volume. The chapters provide an impetus for a study of the problems and stimulate further thinking regarding their resolution.

It is encouraging that in the 1980s the case for emphasizing cultural context in the understanding, treatment, and prevention of mental disorders has been made extensively and persuasively. What is needed now is no longer ideology but actual techniques and methods for our daily work. The chapters in the current volume demonstrate that we are far away from having a perfect recipe for rendering culturally sensitive services; however, the foundations are available for building the needed new approaches. There are numerous case examples that demonstrate that with proper planning, training, and commitment, the cultural context of mental health services can be taken into account in the provision of care. The problem we face, however, is going from general knowledge about culture traditions to specific mental health practices. This is where the disagreements, debates, and arguments begin and where the pragmatists frequently lose interest.

There is little agreement about the specific content and process involved in training mental health professionals to become culturally sensitive. Like many topics, it may be easier to talk about principles and goals than about the implementation of methods. The numerous anecdotes of success and failure and the nascent empirical studies and demonstration projects still await systematization and operational application. There are a number of reasons for the current state of affairs.

First, it is apparent that there is extensive confusion in the use of terminology. Words such as "culture," "ethnicity," "health," "symptoms," "therapy," and so forth are often used quite casually with very different intended meanings. We face the challenge of agreeing to definitions of meanings for these terms so that communication can be improved. Such a task would obviously be tedious and frustrating and the product might not satisfy all of the purists; however, it would be an important beginning and could provide the type of platform necessary for launching successful culturally sensitive practices.

Second, we face problems in measurement. These problems include the usual difficulties of reliability and validity as well as the special problems encountered in cross-cultural research, including back-translation, conceptual equivalence, and scale equivalence. Specific cultural studies become useful for demonstrating issues and problems, but until a systematic international effort is made to address the problems of measurement, it will be difficult for significant advances to be made.

Third, there is little agreement about the nature of therapy and the factors responsible for its successes and failures. These problems are amplified when we cross cultural boundaries. There are hundreds of systems of counseling and psychotherapy that have been developed in the Western world. In addition, every non-Western culture has an indigenous system that emerged from the context of the culture's unique history and development. We know little about the Western systems and even less about the indigenous ones. On the one hand, it is easy to speculate that the potent mediators of change in all therapy and counseling include a variety of factors such as insight, catharsis, hope, guilt reduction, increased information, and reduction of uncertainty. However, without understanding how these forces are mobilized and maintained in different cultural contexts, we face serious problems.

Fourth, we are faced with an enormous challenge from pharmacological treatments now available throughout the world. Pharmacological treatments are powerful and deal with symptoms rapidly and economically. There are, of course, many shortcomings in pharmacological treatments; but, in the face of the complexities of psychotherapy and counseling, these shortcomings are often overlooked and pharmacological treatment is preferred.

Fifth, the economic, political, and social situations in developing nations may not encourage the implementation of culturally sensitive services. Many of the mental health professionals in these countries receive training in Western settings and find it difficult to understand or support indigenous approaches to health care. Further, many of the professionals end up in administrative positions because of the scarcity of trained personnel. Budgets, resources, and facilities become an end in themselves amid the developing country's push for industrialization and economic specialization. Approaches that endorse indigenous ways are often frowned upon as inappropriate. In addition, mental health problems are forced to yield to extensive physical health problems related to poverty, malnutrition, crowding, overpopulation, and limited educational opportunities.

These factors make it difficult to move from ideologies to practice in the delivery of culturally sensitive mental health services. The problems are conceptual, methodological, and pragmatic. Even a well-intentioned mental health professional will have to struggle with the complex realities of each situation.

A NEW DOCTRINE

Amid these problems a new doctrine is emerging that may hold the answer to the stated problems. The most important tenet of the new doctrine is the decentralization of mental health services and their integration with existing general health care services. With the exception of a small group of mental disorders requiring highly specialized care and facilities, most mental health problems could benefit from integration of mental health with other health and/or social service systems in various countries. This tenet may well alter the nature and mission of psychiatry. The tenet favors a multidisciplinary approach in which the behavioral sciences and the humanities may make a significant contribution. The chapters in this volume illustrate how some of the services abiding by this new doctrine can work. They also suggest the need for new types of mental health research.

For example, it would be valuable if cross-cultural comparisons concentrated more frequently on differences within the researcher's own country. A look at changes in time or a comparison of different population groups living in the same location blended with clinical insights and epidemiological estimates of service needs could help both science and those concerned with service development. This does not mean that collaboration across national borders is unnecessary. The validity of findings of cross-cultural research within countries can best be supported by comparison of results with those obtained in cross-cultural work done by researchers using equivalent methods in their own settings and coming together to understand and interpret their findings.

The scarce fiscal resources could be used in more multidisciplinary studies of service delivery of ethnocultural variations in responses to psychotropic drugs, of mental health protective factors among people living in difficult situations, and the role of the family in mediating stress of rapid socioeconomic change.

Also, there have been few studies on attitude formation, behavior modification, and decision making in the developing world. For example, almost nothing is known about the diffusion of health information in urban slums in developing countries. The changes in attitude formation that occur as a result of rapidly changing socioeconomic conditions is another topic deserving attention.

The functioning of services under different socioeconomic conditions is another area of research that needs development. The comparative method of research and the application of mental health to behavioral science and operational research issues may provide particularly useful information. In most countries, such comparisons could be done in the same geographical location.

This book also clearly demonstrates that there is more to mental health programs than treatment of the severely mentally ill. Enlightened mental health programs can make a significant contribution to the definition of health and health care. An important contribution can be made to research methodology stemming from mental health and behavioral sciences applied to issues of mental functioning. There is, finally, a significant contribution mental health programs can make in the process of helping those addressing general health services.

The need to "think culture" in the provision of care, in planning and evaluating services, and in carrying out research and training is a further insight brought out by the chapters of this book. The need for a careful description and evaluation of innovative approaches to the organization of care is another. Rich lessons can be learned from the study of ways in which traditional practitioners handle mental disorder. Reliance on a single method of therapy is clearly not in the best interest of those who suffer. An eclectic or multimodal approach, using every manner of treatment that has been proven useful, has a better chance to help the patient, the family, and the community.

There are both similarities and significant differences between mental disorders in different cultures. Their study can help us to reach conclusions about ways of treatment organization and can increase our understanding of human functioning in health and disease in different cultures. Finally, there are concrete tasks that urgently need to be done, including the already-mentioned concerted efforts to reach a common understanding of terms, a common use of methods that allow comparative study, and a common definition of goals of research and service, goals whose definition and implementation will involve all concerned—the community, individuals (healthy or sick), politicians, scientists, and care providers—in a new, positive, and more powerful alliance.

Author Index

287

Subject Index

About the Authors

Erika Bourguignon is Professor and former Chair of the Department of Anthropology at Ohio State University. She received her Ph.D. in anthropology from Northwestern University. She has conducted field research among the Chippewa Indians of Wisconsin and in Haiti. She is the editor of *Religion, Altered States of Consciousness and Social Change* (1973) and *A World of Women* (198). She is the author of *Possession* (1976) and *Psychological Anthropology* (1979) and, with Lenora Greenbaum, *Diversity and Homogeneity in World Societies* (1973).

Norman G. Dinges (Ph.D., Colorado State University) currently is a Clinical Associate Professor of Psychiatry at the Oregon Health Sciences University and a Senior Postdoctoral Fellow at the Institute on Aging at Portland State University. His research interests include intercultural competence, developmental intervention with Navajo parents and children, cross-ethnic studies of the elderly, and cross-cultural psychotherapy.

Takeo Doi is Director of the National Institute of Mental Health of Japan. His former positions include Professor of Mental Health and Psychiatry at the University of Tokyo, Visiting Scientist at the (U.S.) National Institute of Mental Health, and Fellow of the Menninger School of Psychiatry. He received his degree from the University of Tokyo School of Medicine in 1942.

Juris G. Draguns is a clinical psychologist (Ph.D., University of Rochester). For the past twenty years he has been actively involved in cross-cultural research on manifestations of psychopathology, personality variables, and values. He has also been interested in cultural variations in the counseling and psychotherapeutic process. He is coeditor of the *Handbook of Cross-Cultural Psychology,*

Volume 6: Psychopathology and of *Counseling Across Cultures*, associate editor of the *Journal of Cross-Cultural Psychology*, and author of numerous book chapters and articles in psychological psychiatric and anthropological journals. He is Professor of Psychology at Pennsylvania State University, where he teaches graduate courses in cultural psychology, psychopathology personality theory, and clinical assessment.

G. Allen German is Professor of Psychiatry at the University of Western Australia. He is also a consultant psychiatrist for the Sir Charles Gairdner Hospital, the Royal Perth Hospital, and the King Edward Memorial Hospital, all in Perth, Western Australia. He was previously Foundation Professor of Psychiatry, Makerere University, Uganda. He graduated from the University of Aberdeen with a degree in medicine in 1958, and received his graduate training in psychiatry at the Maudsley Hospital, London.

Howard N. Higginbotham received a doctorate in clinical psychology from the University of Hawaii in 1979. He then cofounded and directed New Zealand's first professional community psychology program at Waikato in Hamilton for three years before returning as a research fellow to the East-West Center, Institute of Culture and Communication. His Ph.D. research involved a survey of psychiatric resources in Southeast Asia and the problem of culture accommodation in mental health care. A complete description of his survey findings were recently published in a volume entitled *Third World Challenge to Psychiatry* (University of Hawaii Press, 1984).

Harriet P. Lefley is Associate Professor and Director of the Cross-Cultural Training Institute of the Department of Psychiatry, University of Miami School of Medicine. She is also Director of Research, Planning, and Evaluation of the New Horizons Community Mental Health Center, formerly the University of Miami-Jackson Memorial Medical Center Community Mental Health Center.

Madeleine Leininger is Professor of Nursing and Anthropology and Director of the Center of Health Research at the College of Nursing, Wayne State University. She is also a teacher, researcher, and consultant in transcultural health and nursing. Her past positions include Distinguished Visiting Sorrell Professor of Nursing, Troy State University System, and Dean and Professor of Nursing and Adjunct Professor in Anthropology, College of Nursing, University of Utah. Her publications include *Basic Concepts in Psychiatric Nursing* (1960), *Transcultural Nursing: Theories, Concepts and Practices* (1978), and *Transcultural Theory* (in press).

Spero M. Manson (Ph.D., University of Minnesota) is an Associate Professor of Psychiatry and Director of Social Psyciatric Research at the Oregon Health Sciences University in Portland, Oregon. He also holds the position of Associate Professor at the Institute on Aging at Portland State University. A medical and cultural anthropologist, he has conducted mental health research on depression among Southeast Asian refugees and black and American Indian elderly, and adaptations to problematic life events and civil commitment of American Indians.

Thomas W. Maretzki is Professor of Anthropology at the University of Hawaii. He holds faculty appointments in the Department of Anthropology, Faculty of Social Sciences, and in the Department of Allied Medical Sciences, John A. Burns School of Medicine. He directs a postdoctoral training program in clinically applied medical anthropology, currently concentrating on mental health problems in primary medicine. He has been active as a cultural psychiatry teaching and research consultant in Indonesia since 1966.

Anthony J. Marsella is Professor, Department of Psychology, University of Hawaii, and Director, World Health Organization Psychiatric Research Center, The Queen's Medical Center, Honolulu, Hawaii. He received his Ph.D. in clinical psychology from Penn State University in 1968. He is a former Fulbright Professor to the Philippines and an NIMH Culture and Mental Health Research Scholar. His primary research interest is in the area of cross-cultural psychopathology. He has published six books and more than sixty chapters and journal articles.

Beatrice Medicine (Ph.D., University of Wisconsin) is currently at the Department of Anthropology at California State University at Northridge. As a cultural and medical anthropologist, her research and writing have emphasized the contemporary condition of American Indians and Alaska Natives. Her special interests involve the mental health of Indian women, an ethnographic approach to the study of drinking and sobriety, and life history work of selected Indian elders. In 1983 she was the recipient of the Outstanding Woman of Color award presented in Washington, D.C.

Paul B. Pedersen is Professor of Education and Chair of the Counseling Program at Syracuse University. He has taught in Asian universities for six years and directed an NIMH training program in Hawaii for four years. He has published more than a hundred books, articles, and chapters on aspects of cross-cultural counseling and communication. He has been President of the Society for Intercultural Education Training and Research and has been active in promoting intercultural counseling through both the American Psychological Association and the American Association for Counseling and Development.

Raymond Prince is Professor, Department of Psychiatry, McGill University. Since 1982, he has been Editor of *Transcultural Psychiatric Research Review*. His current research deals with culture, stress, and illness, particularly coronary heart disease.

Norman Sartorius was appointed Director of the Division of Mental Health, World Health Organization, in January 1977. He joined WHO in 1967 as a consultant; he worked in Southeast Asia and other regions, and later assumed charge of the program of epidemiological and social psychiatry. He has been principal investigator of the International Pilot Study on Schizophrenia, the International Study on Depression, and other projects. He has published over a hundred articles in scientific journals and is coauthor of several books. He also holds the Chair of Transcultural Psychiatry at the Medical School of the University of Zagreb and is an Associate of the Faculty of the School of Public Health at Johns Hopkins University. He is a member of the editorial boards of a number of scientific journals and honorary member of many professional and learned associations.

Joseph E. Trimble (Ph.D., University of Oklahoma) is an Associate Professor of Psychology at Western Washington University, Bellingham, Washington. His research interests include the study of adaptive strategies of culturally diverse groups to life-threatening and problematic life events, use of behavior-cognitive mediated strategies in mental health, and substance abuse intervention and prevention. He has served on a number of agencies and committees of the National Institute of Mental Health, National Institute of Alcohol Abuse and Alcoholism, National Institute of Drug Abuse, and the American Psychological Association.